A DELICATE BALANCE

Living Successfully with Chronic Illness

A DELICATE BALANCE

Living Successfully with Chronic Illness

SUSAN MILSTREY WELLS

Foreword by

KATHERINE MORLAND HAMMITT
President, Sjogren's Syndrome Foundation

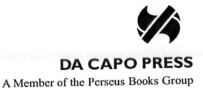

DA CAPO PRESS
A Member of the Perseus Books Group

The excerpt from the poem, "We're Fine, Just Fine, or, You'll Be Astonished When I'm Gone, You Rascal, You," on page 142 is from *There's Always Another Windmill* by Ogden Nash. ©1967 by Ogden Nash. By permission of Little, Brown and Company. Also, international rights, ©1968 by Ogden Nash. Reprinted by permission of Curtis Brown, Ltd.

The quote on page 87 is from *Manifesto for a New Medicine: Your Guide to Healing Partnerships and the Wise Use of Alternative Therapies* by James S. Gordon (Addison-Wesley, Reading, Massachusetts, 1996). ©1996 James S. Gordon; used with permission.

The information in this book is based on the experiences and research of the author. This material is for informational purposes only and should not be construed as prescribing information for individual patients. The author and publisher assume no responsibility for any treatment undertaken by the practitioner with individual patients. Companies, interventions, and products are mentioned without bias to increase your knowledge only.

A CIP catalog record for this book is available from the Library of Congress. ISBN 0-7382-0323-X

Published by Da Capo Press, A member of the Perseus Books Group

Find us on the World Wide Web at http://www.perseusbooks.com

Books published by the Perseus Books Group are available at special discounts for bulk purchases in the United States by corporations, institutions, and other organizations. For more information, please contact the Special Markets Department at the Perseus Books Group, 11 Cambridge Center, Cambridge, MA 02142, or call (617) 252-5298, (800) 255-1514 or e-mail special.markets@perseusbooks.com.

First paperback printing, June 2000

To the late Sally Sutta,
my favorite Aunt, who knew it wasn't all in her head

and to my husband, Glenn Wells, and my son, Raymond Milstrey,
without whose unflagging love, patience, and ability to make me
laugh, I never would have realized my dream

CONTENTS

FOREWORD

Susan Milstrey Wells has touched my life and will touch yours as well. Those of us who suffer from a chronic illness struggle to find ways to make our lives easier and better. Illness profoundly changes our lives as well as the lives of those around us. Whether you are the one who is ill or whether someone you know and care about is ill, this book will embrace you with understanding and compassion and bring you a wealth of practical information.

Physical symptoms might differ, but the emotional stresses that make us human create problems we all share. I have Sjogren's (pronounced *SHOW-grins*) syndrome, often called "a disease that doesn't show." Sufferers are told, "But you look just fine!" However, like many chronic illnesses that "don't show," Sjogren's has devastating consequences for those of us who have it, who also have the unique problem of convincing others that we really are not well. Our quality of life is radically altered since we spend our very limited energy searching for answers and for doctors who will listen, redefining how we relate to our friends and loved ones, and learning how to live with the physical pain, fatigue, and disabilities of a disease that we didn't ask for and was not in our life plan.

Susan brings a highly experienced background to this book. She has been a writer and journalist for twenty years, with special expertise in the fields of mental health, education, and social policy. But just as importantly, she has several chronic illnesses herself, much like many of those she writes about. Sjogren's syndrome, for example, can occur as a single disease or may accompany other autoimmune disorders, such as lupus and rheumatoid arthritis.

Susan reminds us how difficult it is for people with a chronic illness to live a normal life in a society that judges us severely on the basis of health and productivity. The relationships we forge with our doctors, employers and co-workers, and friends and family have a vital impact on our adjustment to our illness, ability to cope, and personal growth. For example, because they live with a chronically ill mother and hear me talk with others who call to share their stories of coping with a chronic illness, my own children, Kelsey and Kenneth, have developed a rare sensitivity to and caring feeling for others. They have had to suffer with me, sharing the fear and questions that a chronic illness brings. Yet, they have grown and learned from its restrictions to become a real source of strength and support for me, and I'm sure they will be for others in the years to come. As a family, we have learned to share a deep appreciation for life, recognize its fragility, and accept who we are in a world that does not often reward those who are different. Our experience is teaching us a lifelong lesson that we can apply whether our struggle is with chronic illness or something else.

I like Susan's use of the word *journey* in the title of chapter 1 and throughout the book. Chronic illness is indeed a journey, fraught with hazards, detours, breakdowns, and even lost ways, but it also offers new routes and views and progress toward our hoped-for destination of health and fulfillment. *A Delicate Balance* provides an excellent guide and support for this journey, from finding the elusive diagnosis to handling others' reactions to our illness, building good doctor–patient relationships, searching for treatments and answers, balancing work and illness, discovering what makes us feel well, and learning how to rise above it all and obtain that delicate balance of living well with a chronic illness in a healthy world.

Susan encourages us to be our own best advocates by understanding our illness and educating ourselves. She mentions the importance of my experience of participating in a support group. As three-term president of and long-term volunteer with the Sjogren's Syndrome Foundation, I have learned that together we can accomplish so much more than we can as individuals. As we talk with one another, learning about our disease through the foundation's newsletters and publications, join together to present our needs, and see our needs addressed in research and recognized publicly and medically, we are empowered and find we are not alone. We can learn from one another, and we can share our pain and joy with one another.

This book helps us to do these things too. I felt I came to know the people Susan interviewed as friends, as people who face many of the same frustrations and obstacles—whether in dealing with Sjogren's syndrome, fibromyalgia, lupus, multiple sclerosis, interstitial cystitis, chronic fatigue syndrome, or any other chronic illness. I felt enriched by those who were willing to share the details of their lives. Then I could say, "Yes, I know, that's me, too" or "What a good approach or tip! I'd like to try that." They offered a way of life that is not only possible but full of hope.

A Delicate Balance reaches out not only to people with chronic illness and their friends and family, but also to a much wider audience. Doctors and students of psychology will gain a better understanding of what it's like to have a chronic illness. In fact, everyone has much to gain from the profound philosophy of life that is presented in the pages of this book.

Katherine Morland Hammitt
President, Sjogren's Syndrome Foundation

PREFACE

Both my teenage son and my best friend of thirty years became ill the year I started to write this book. What seemed at first to be a cruel twist of fate reenergized me to move forward with a project that now seemed more important than ever.

I learned from both of them. Because I fear that giving in to my health problems might mean giving up I push through the pain and fatigue, but my son intuitively knows how to listen to his body and to rest when he feels tired. My friend is in the early stages of an illness that has yet to be named. Talking to her made me realize that I have reached an uneasy acceptance with chronic health problems, but I also discovered I still have a way to go.

I have accepted that there is no known cause or cure for the multiple illnesses I have. Knowing that there is not a magic pill that will take away my fatigue and my pain, I can focus on learning how to make myself feel better. And I accept the fact that, though I have an innate drive to be certain about everything, there is much about my health problems I will never fully understand.

However, I have a more difficult time coming to terms with the impact my health problems have on my family and friends and on my career. My husband and I work hard to make our marriage succeed within the constraints that chronic illness imposes. Writing, my chosen profession, feels like more than a career. Being a writer is *who I am*. Learning to put work in its proper perspective is an ongoing balancing act for me.

Most of all, I struggle with my self-image. The ability to work hard, be productive, and handle multiple stressors with aplomb are highly prized traits in today's society. Women in particular seem to juggle numerous roles with equanimity. I sometimes think of myself as "defective," an imposter in a healthy world.

In looking for resources to help me cope, I scanned the health and self-help sections of bookstores and, more recently, began perusing the Internet. Though there is a good deal of information available on living with chronic illness, I didn't find exactly what I was looking for. I wanted information that was

- *comprehensive*, focusing not on a specific illness but on the experience of living with chronic disease,
- *consumer-oriented*, based on the real-life experiences of individuals living successfully with chronic illness, and
- *concrete*, offering practical advice based on personal experience.

When multiple health problems began to take their toll in recent years, I turned to what I know best. I've been a journalist for half my life, and gathering information by talking to people isn't just my livelihood—it is the way I organize and understand my world.

When I started talking to others about their experiences with chronic illness, I discovered that I am not alone. I learned that my doubts, fears, and grief are normal, and that laughter is good medicine for pain. I marveled at individuals' passionate struggles and quiet acceptance, and I uncovered some practical tips for healthy living. Like many, I had spent years in what felt like a desperate search for *the* answer. I realized that some of us find it, but most of us don't.

Yet, in spite of, or perhaps because of, the lack of a cure for our illnesses, we start to heal. We begin taking better care of ourselves when we accept the fact that we're sick and believe that we deserve to be well. Finding a delicate balance between giving in to our disease and thinking we have to conquer it, we learn to accept what life sends our way. This is a good way to live, with or without chronic illness.

My conversations with patients, providers, and family members gave me both the validation I was seeking and the information I needed to live a healthier life with chronic disease. They also taught me much about myself. *A Delicate Balance* is a gift to myself that I am privileged to share.

ACKNOWLEDGMENTS

There are many people without whom this book would not have been possible. First and foremost, I owe an enormous debt of gratitude to the women and men, named and unnamed, who openly shared intimate and painful details of their lives in the hope that others might benefit from their experiences. They taught me much about living successfully with chronic illness and about myself. My thanks go also to the family members and friends, and to the professionals in the fields of medicine, social work, and disability, whose insights and knowledge corroborate the patient's perspective.

Special thanks go to the following individuals for their unique contributions to this project and to my life: to my parents, Nedwin and Marjorie Emerson and the late Elaine Parry, and to my brothers, Stephen Emerson and Scott Emerson, and their families, for loving and encouraging me; to my husband, Glenn Wells, for giving me physical, financial, and emotional support and never-ending love and for compiling the endnotes; to my son, Raymond Milstrey, for always finding the positive in life and never failing to make me laugh; to Laurie Nugent, for thirty years of unconditional friendship; to Rita Earle, who wisely suggested that writing this book was an important way for me to heal; to Sonia Boffa, for believing I could do it; to Gail Metzger and her sister Laurie Burns, for transcribing the bulk of my interview tapes for a song; to the Rev. Christopher M. Dillon, for bringing Rita, Sonia, Gail, and me together, and for guiding me in my growing faith; to Dr. Richard A. Brown, for believing me when I said I didn't feel well; to Dr. Daniel J. Clauw, Dr. James S. Gordon, and Mark Fishelman, for reviewing selected portions of the text; to Sharon Ross, for her insightful comments about the text and about me; to Mary Anne Saathoff, for providing excellent leads; to Alexis Stegemann of the Sjogren's Syndrome Foundation, for putting me in touch with the right people; to Deirdre Oakley and to the reference librarians at the Shenendehowa Public Library in Clifton Park, New York, for patiently answering my many questions; to Meg Gallien, for editing the page proofs with a trained and caring eye; to my editor, Frank Darmstadt, for gently encouraging me to share more of myself; and last but not least to Pauline Bartel, teacher, mentor, colleague, and friend, for helping me conceive this project, and for holding my hand during the labor and delivery. Without her unwavering belief in me and my work, *A Delicate Balance* never would have been born.

A DELICATE BALANCE

Living Successfully with Chronic Illness

INTRODUCTION

Chronic illness doesn't come with an instruction manual. I know that I have Sjogren's syndrome, an autoimmune disease that results in dry eyes and dry mouth; fibromyalgia, a condition marked by diffuse musculoskeletal pain and fatigue; and interstitial cystitis, a chronic inflammation of the bladder. But I knew very little about how others lived with these and similar diseases, including chronic fatigue syndrome, lupus, Lyme disease, multiple sclerosis, and inflammatory bowel disease. Because these diseases are unfamiliar to both the general public and professionals, the National Organization of Rare Disorders (NORD) in New Fairfield, Connecticut, considers many of these illnesses "back-of-the-textbook" diseases. The symptoms of most of these illnesses are largely invisible; pain and fatigue are hard to see. Further, the course of these diseases fluctuates from day to day and year to year, and they run the gamut from mild to seriously disabling.

Relying on my training as a journalist, I interviewed more than three dozen women and men throughout the United States and Canada to learn how they manage the pain, uncertainty, and fear of living with ongoing health problems. I met a remarkable group of people whose stories I am proud to share in the pages that follow. We laughed and cried together, and I learned some important lessons from each one of my new friends.

I also spoke with family members and friends of people who are sick to understand firsthand how our experiences affect the people we love. Then I asked more than a dozen professionals, from social workers to physicians to disability advocates, to explain in more detail the physical and emotional impact of living with chronic illness. In addition, I scoured books, research articles, and on-line resources for clues about the causes of certain illnesses and the newest theories on treatment. In sharing this information, I hope to give back some of the validation, insight, and support that was given to me. *A Delicate Balance* is the book I wish someone had given me when I first became sick.

MAKING THE JOURNEY

Getting sick is the beginning of a journey toward understanding, accepting, and healing. The steps we take along the way form the framework for this book.

Chapter 1, "Beginning the Journey: The Search for a Diagnosis," examines some of the reasons why a chronic disease may be hard to diagnose and looks at the self-doubt and social stigma that comes with having unnamed symptoms. We can easily get caught up in the search for an accurate diagnosis; this chapter reminds us that we can begin to take care of ourselves even before our illness has a name.

Accepting the fact that we are sick requires that we believe in ourselves. We might discount what we feel, however, when told repeatedly that our symptoms are "all in our head." Chapter 2, "A Stumbling Block: Is My Illness Really 'All in My Head'?" examines the delicate balance between our physical and emotional health. Understanding that what we think can affect how we feel may lead us to believe that we caused our illnesses; this chapter reminds us about the important distinction between blame and responsibility.

Knowledge about our physical and emotional health can help us choose an appropriate health care provider. Chapter 3, "Finding a Health Care Partner," examines how technology and managed-care regulations have altered the doctor–patient relationship. Selecting a capable and caring health care partner is critical for those of us living with chronic disease; this chapter reminds us that it is both our right and our responsibility to do so.

Once we have named our disease and found a health care partner, we turn our attention to treatment. Chapter 4, "Now What? The Search for Treatments," examines attitudes and beliefs about traditional and alternative treatments, and explores how individuals evaluate the effectiveness and safety of suggested remedies. This chapter reminds us to have a healthy skepticism about alleged "cures" that seem too good to be true. We explore some of the therapies that help us get better in chapter 5, "Discovering What Makes Us Feel Well."

The emotional fallout of chronic illness can be as devastating as the physical disease. Chronic illness isolates us, and we need to grieve our losses. Chapter 6, "From Denial to Acceptance and Back Again," reminds us that we must confront our negative emotions before we can let them go.

Chapter 7, "How to Be Sick in a Healthy World," looks at the effect of chronic illness on personal relationships. Our family and friends experience many of the same losses we do. They want to help but may feel frustrated that they can't make us better. Having chronic illness in the family can threaten the best of relationships; this chapter shows that it also can make them stronger.

The physical, emotional, and social consequences of chronic illness intersect at the point where our health problems impact our ability to earn a living. Chapter 8, "Changing the Way We Look at Work," examines the impact of our health on our work. To protect our health, some of us choose to become self-employed or leave work altogether, living on disability or dwindling savings. We may feel diminished and devalued by these changes; this chapter reminds us that we can define ourselves by who we *are*, not by what we *do*.

Finally, chapter 9, "The Gift of Chronic Illness," looks beyond our daily struggles with chronic disease. Life with ongoing health problems is thankless and difficult, yet many of us find ways to turn limitations into opportunities. This chapter suggests that chronic illness can reveal the path to a healthier life.

It is my hope that all who are affected by chronic disease will benefit from this information. For those of us who are ill, chronic illness sets us apart. But when we read about the experiences of others, we realize that we are not alone and that healing is available to all of us, regardless of our disease.

Chronic illness often is unspeakable, either because of the intimate nature of our symptoms or our fears of being considered hypochondriacs or malingerers. But when they read about our fears, frustrations, and needs, our family, friends, and colleagues may come to better understand our struggles. And when we listen to them, we will be more aware of their concerns.

Finally, I hope this book will guide those who care for us. We turn to doctors, therapists, healers, and clergy in our search for better health. The more we understand one another's roles in dealing with chronic illness, the better able we are to form effective partnerships.

I often find myself thinking about my paternal grandmother, Grandma Rose, who had a philosophy about life that makes me smile. No matter the problem, she would say with confidence, "Oh well, as long as you have your health." I smile because I do have enough health to raise my teenage son, nurture my marriage, and make money as a writer and editor. Indeed, I often have said that my health problems are not life threatening. Rather, they are "quality of life threatening."

A Delicate Balance is about a search for quality. We need to gain enough information to manage our physical symptoms successfully, but we also have to learn to live with a certain amount of ambiguity and uncertainty. Striving for a delicate balance between work and play, rest and activity, relationships and solitude, and grief and joy, we come to accept our limitations and rejoice in our gifts.

Living successfully with chronic illness takes patience, humor, knowledge, support, and time. I hope that we can take time to find knowledge, seek support, reflect with humor, and be patient with ourselves as we travel this road together.

BEGINNING THE JOURNEY

The Search for a Diagnosis

A journey of a thousand miles must begin with a single step.
LAO-TZU

Being sick is hard work. When pain and fatigue become part of our every-day lives, we need extra energy for routine tasks, such as showering or making dinner. Many days, that leaves little energy for our new job of being a person with a chronic disease. One of our first and most important tasks is to figure out why we don't feel well. In this chapter, we'll explore why it is so important for us to get a diagnosis, and we'll discuss the great lengths to which we go in order to do so. We'll examine the vagaries of the diagnostic process, which help explain why it can take months or even years before we know what is wrong with us. Finally, we'll consider the fact that our need to have a definitive diagnosis may be less important than our need to learn how to take care of ourselves. We can only begin to get better when we balance self-knowledge with self-care.

SEEKING THE DIAGNOSTIC HANDLE

Chronic illness has a dramatic impact on our lives, whether it begins suddenly or builds gradually. Like a piece of bad news we try to forget, the knowledge that we are sick bubbles to the surface unbidden. Uncertainty, fear, and anxiety often accompany the physical symptoms, and we struggle to find a way to describe what is happening to us.

Clinical social worker and trauma specialist Patricia A. Fennell, president of Albany Health Management Associates, Inc., and senior clinical consultant to the Capital Region Sleep/Wake Disorder Clinic in Albany, New York, calls the search to name our disease "the battle of the 'diagnostic handle.' As individuals, we categorize our experiences to help us understand our reality, and language is key to doing that."

A diagnosis validates our reality. Without a symbol to describe our experiences, Fennell suggests, we may deny that there is anything wrong with us, doubt the reality of our own perceptions, blame ourselves for being lazy or crazy, and meet with disbelief from family, friends, and even our doctors. Looking back on the years in which I was becoming increasingly sick, I remember being frustrated at my lack of stamina, frightened about my future, and confused about the fact that no one could find anything wrong with me. With all my heart, I wanted to be well, not only for myself but also for my son, who was very young when his father and I divorced.

Desperation

An intense and immediate change in our health makes us desperate for answers and for relief. Eileen knows exactly when she became sick. "It was the day after Thanksgiving, ten and a half years ago," says Eileen, age forty-nine, who developed an apparent urinary tract infection that never went away. In pain and needing to use a bathroom frequently, she found it difficult to concentrate on her job as a fourth-grade teacher. Her search for a diagnosis consumed the next five years of her life.

"I went crazy the first year I became sick," Eileen says. "My whole life was spent going to doctors." In between medical appointments, she started reading about urological disorders, and she began to suspect that she had interstitial cystitis, a chronic inflammation of the bladder. To fill the vacuum left by lack of a diagnosis, many of us with a chronic illness conduct our own research, a topic we'll touch on further in later chapters. However, none of the doctors Eileen saw was able to confirm a diagnosis. Tired of making the rounds, she tried to ignore ongoing bladder pain for another year before becoming "desperate" enough to begin seeing doctors again.

Eileen's desperation may have led her to decide on a procedure she didn't need. Her gynecologist suggested a hysterectomy because he believed this would make room for her bladder to expand. So, at age forty-two, with no children, Eileen had removed a large but healthy uterus and one ovary. "All that time I kept saying the pain was in my bladder," Eileen says. And, indeed, her bladder symptoms became worse after the surgery. Finally, five years after she first became sick, a urologist diagnosed Eileen with interstitial cystitis. Urgency, frequency, and pain are the principal symptoms of this disorder. According to the Interstitial Cystitis Association (ICA), nearly half a million Americans may have this disease, the majority of them women. Accurate prevalence rates are difficult to determine because researchers often use different methods to define the disease.[1] More information about national organizations like the ICA that are mentioned throughout this book can be found in the resources at the end of the book.

Ken Henderson had a similar experience. In early 1994, Ken, age fifty, started having pains just below the left side of his rib cage. His doctor thought it was referred pain from the gallbladder, which is in the same position on the right side. Referred pain is pain caused in one part of the body but felt in another. Though an ultrasound didn't reveal any problems with the gallbladder, Ken says, "My doctor thought that removing it would straighten me out." But instead, the surgery only exacerbated Ken's pain, and a pathology report indicated that his gallbladder had been perfectly healthy. Ken subsequently was diagnosed with fibromyalgia, a condition marked by diffuse musculoskeletal pain and fatigue. Today, Ken is more resentful than angry about the unnecessary surgery. He says, "I'd sure like to have my gallbladder back."

According to Dr. Don L. Goldenberg, chief of rheumatology and director of the Arthritis/Fibromyalgia Center at Newton-Wellesley Hospital in Newton, Massachusetts, fibromyalgia is the second most frequent diagnosis made by rheumatologists, doctors who specialize in treating arthritis and other disorders of the joints, muscles, and connective tissues.[2] For reasons that are not yet clearly understood, fibromyalgia is ten times more common in women than in men. Dr. Goldenberg estimates that six to ten million Americans, including children, have fibromyalgia. Worldwide, fibromyalgia affects 2 to 6 percent of the population in countries that have compiled these data.[3]

Though fibromyalgia is not degenerative, the disease can be highly disabling. Researchers at a Swedish rheumatology clinic measured the perceived coping abilities of fifty women with fibromyalgia, forty-seven women with rheumatoid arthritis, and forty-two women with systemic lupus erythematosus (lupus). Although all of the groups indicated some lack of ability to manage their symptoms and control pain, the women with fibromyalgia perceived they had less control over their disease.[4]

Fear and Uncertainty

When the onset of chronic disease is more gradual, we may live for months or even years with a foreboding sense that something is terribly wrong with us. Kathy Hammitt, president of the Sjogren's Syndrome Foundation, had swollen parotid (salivary) and lymph glands and low-grade fevers from the age of twenty-six on. Now forty-four, she pursued a diagnosis off and on for years, reactivating her search each time she was troubled by a new symptom. After her first child was born, Kathy became much worse. Weak, feverish, and in pain, she gave up her job as news producer for a television network affiliate. She was told she had everything from gland infections to lymphoma, a cancer of the lymph system.

Six years after she began actively seeking a diagnosis, Kathy learned she has Sjogren's syndrome, an autoimmune disease marked by inflammation and eventual destruction of the body's exocrine (moisture-producing) glands. Painfully dry eyes resulting in blurred vision, burning and itching, and intolerance to bright light are a hallmark of Sjogren's syndrome. Lack of saliva may cause difficulties in talking and swallowing, as well as an increase in tooth decay and gum disease. Once thought to be rare, the prevalence of Sjogren's syndrome is reported to be 1 to 3 percent of the general population in countries that have gathered these statistics.[5] According to the Sjogren's Syndrome Foundation, the disease strikes between two and four million Americans, many of whom go undiagnosed. Nine out of ten individuals with Sjogren's syndrome are women. Because of the predominance of women with autoimmune diseases—those in which the body mistakes its own cells as foreign invaders—physicians and scientists are beginning to study the role of female hormones in the development of these illnesses.

Like Kathy, I too have Sjogren's syndrome. In my sophomore year in high school, I spent a month in the hospital with swollen glands and a fever of indeterminate origin. This was in the days before managed care, so the length of my stay may not be indicative of the seriousness of the problem. Nevertheless, my doctors were concerned enough about the possibility of Hodgkin's disease, a malignant disorder of the lymph system, to biopsy one of my glands. The biopsy was negative, and I returned to school after a three-month absence.

In the years that followed, I was plagued by frequent upper respiratory, vaginal, and urinary tract infections, periodic swelling of my salivary glands, and unremitting fatigue. However, I was in my midthirties before a doctor tested me for evidence of autoimmunity and began to consider that I might have Sjogren's syndrome. Even then, it was several more years before he could confirm a diagnosis. In the meantime, I lived in an ambiguous state between no diagnosis and multiple possibilities. I wondered if I were imagining my symptoms or if the doctors were missing evidence of a serious and potentially fatal disease. Looking back, I recall feeling that my fear and confusion would never end. I didn't start to feel better physically or emotionally until I had some concrete answers.

Shock

Sometimes an illness that seems to begin suddenly actually has been developing slowly over the years. When one of his friends died unexpectedly, Daniel, age forty-six, decided to get a checkup. He had not been to a doctor in fifteen years. A routine physical showed evidence of lesions on the brain, and within months he was diagnosed with multiple sclerosis, a progressive disease of the central nervous system that destroys scattered patches of myelin (the protective covering of nerve fibers) in the brain and spinal cord. Symptoms of multiple sclerosis range from numbness and tingling to incontinence and paralysis. According to the National Multiple Sclerosis Society, 250,000 to 350,000 individuals in the United States have the disease, 70 percent of them women. Multiple sclerosis is one of the most common central nervous system diseases in young adults; an estimated 2.5 million people worldwide have this disorder, according to the International Federation of Multiple Sclerosis Societies.

The diagnosis was a "tremendous shock," Daniel says, but in retrospect he can identify early warning signs: partial loss of vision in his left eye, unexpected weakness, and periodic episodes when he would have to catch himself from tripping.

Denial

Fear that we may be seriously ill sometimes causes us to delay seeking answers. We may find it easier to deny that we are sick. "I started having afternoon runs to the bathroom, but tolerated that for a few months because I was scared to do anything about it," says Linda Webb, age forty-five. "Like many people, I didn't want to know what was wrong because it might be terrible." Linda sought medical help when she noticed blood in her stool. Examination by a gastroenterologist, a physician trained in the management of digestive system disorders, revealed that Linda had ulcerative proctitis, a type of inflammatory bowel disease confined to the rectum. According to the National Institutes of Health, 0.1 percent of the U.S. population, or as many as five hundred thousand people, have inflammatory disorders of the small and large intestine that are marked by abdominal pain, diarrhea, and weight loss. Worldwide prevalence rates range from 0.01 to 0.08 percent, reflecting the role of such risk factors as genetics, environment, and personal health habits.[6] Women have a slightly higher risk of having inflammatory bowel diso.. ; than do men.

Linda survived the prediagnosis period in part by minimizing her symptoms, particularly at work. "I kept saying, 'You can pull out of this,'" she notes. She considers herself to be "a very self-controlled, disciplined person who will leave no stone unturned in a quest to be perfect." Like Linda, I too would often tell myself that I had no reason to feel so poorly, yet, at the same time, I wondered if I would ever feel well again.

Particularly when our illness begins at an early age, we may learn to minimize our symptoms so well that we begin to think they are normal. Sally, age thirty-one, first became sick when she was thirteen. She frequently missed school with various viruses and infections and was often so tired she would fall asleep visiting friends. She made it through college but nearly had to drop out of graduate school because of extended illness. Sally and her family thought she just was prone to being sick. When, at age twenty-four, she received a diagnosis of chronic fatigue syndrome, Sally was amazed to discover she had a number of symptoms that she had never connected to being sick, such as pain in her arms and legs. "I never even thought of mentioning these things to a doctor because they were so continual in my life, I just assumed other people had them too." According to trauma specialist Patricia Fennell, it is not uncommon for people with chronic fatigue syndrome and other diseases that are not yet socially acceptable to deny their symptoms in an effort to continue their daily lives.[7]

Chronic fatigue syndrome is a disorder characterized by debilitating fatigue of unknown cause. According to the Chronic Fatigue and Immune Dysfunction Syndrome (CFIDS) Association of America, two hundred thousand to five hundred thousand adults in the United States have chronic fatigue syndrome. Children and adolescents also have this disorder, though prevalence studies for these groups have not been done. Women are three to seven times more likely than men to be diagnosed with chronic fatigue syndrome. The CFIDS Association bases its figures on conservative estimates by the federal Centers for Disease Control; some patients and advocates criticize the number as being too low. Journalist Hillary Johnson, author of *Osler's Web: Inside the Labyrinth of the Chronic Fatigue Syndrome Epidemic* and herself a patient, suggests that as many as two million people may be afflicted.[8] Differences in theoretical conceptualizations of what constitutes chronic fatigue syndrome may account, in part, for diverse prevalence rates, researchers theorize.[9] Despite official criteria for diagnosing both chronic fatigue syndrome and fibromyalgia, there is considerable controversy in the medical community about the existence of these diseases. We'll examine this topic later in this chapter.

Like Sally, I suffered with symptoms without knowing they might be signs of disease. When I complained to my rheumatologist about diffuse pain throughout my body, and he suspected that I might have fibromyalgia, he asked me if I felt rested when I woke up in the morning. I looked at him in surprise; it hadn't even occurred to me that other people didn't feel tired when they woke up. Research has shown that some people with fibromyalgia have an abnormal sleep pattern marked by interruptions in deep sleep.[10] As we'll see later in this chapter, fibromyalgia often accompanies other rheumatic diseases, such as Sjogren's syndrome.

Denying our symptoms may be something we learn to do at a young age. Miryam Williamson, age sixty, chronicled her experiences with fibromyalgia in her book, *Fibromyalgia: A Comprehensive Approach*. She told me she first remembers feeling pain in her legs at the age of five. "My mother said, 'Everybody has pains,' and I took that very literally to mean that everybody is in pain all the time." She stopped complaining. In her twenties, the pain in her hands was so bad that she used tape instead of safety pins to fasten her baby's diaper. She received a diagnosis of fibromyalgia on October 2, 1993, when she was fifty-seven years old. Even then, Miryam says, "I still didn't know that pain was not a normal condition for people."

Self-Doubt

When we look good but feel terrible and no one can tell us what's wrong, we begin to think we are lazy, or, worse, just plain crazy. "If you're hurting, you know something's wrong," Ken Henderson says. "But after a couple of doctors tell you they can't find anything, you begin to doubt your own sanity." Often, we blame ourselves for some perceived weakness of character.

At various times before she was diagnosed with lupus, thirty-three-year-old Kelly was told she needed to sleep less, lose weight, and exercise more. "My mother said I always required a lot of sleep, so I just thought I was lazy," Kelly says. Systemic lupus erythematosus or lupus is an inflammatory, autoimmune disease that affects various parts of the body, including the skin, joints, blood, and kidneys. According to the Lupus Foundation of America, approximately 1.4 to 2.0 million Americans have this potentially life-threatening disease, 90 percent of them women. Lupus, which means "wolf," is so called because sufferers get a characteristic butterfly-shaped rash across their cheeks and the bridge of their nose that is said to give them a "wolflike" appearance.

Author Linda Hanner suggests that when we lack a diagnosis, we become focused on proving that we really are sick.[11] This struck a chord with me. Before my diagnoses, I put what little energy I had left after working full-time and caring for my son into seeking outside validation that something was wrong with me. Trying to appear sick so doctors will believe us inevitably makes us feel worse, and we end up looking like the hypochondriacs that we know we're not.

"We had a speaker at one of our lupus meetings who said the psychological profile of a lupus patient is that of a hypochondriac," says Jeri, who served as president of her local Lupus Foundation of America chapter. "When you have all these funny little things happening, you're always checking them out. You wonder, 'Is this another symptom? Is it something important? Is this a trend I should keep an eye on?' " Looking back, Jeri, age fifty-two, recognizes a lot of clues leading up to her diagnosis of lupus. She battled oral ulcers, skin lesions, arthritis, and fatigue for more than a decade before a rheumatologist pieced the puzzle together.

Frustration

Lacking any kind of validation, we may stop looking for it altogether. "I'd go as long as two years without seeing a doctor because I was sick and tired of being told that my problems were all in my head," Dulce says. Numerous doctors she consulted over the years told Dulce they could find no physical reasons for her pain, fatigue, and cognitive problems. Raised to believe that only "sissies" complained of pain, Dulce decided to live with her discomfort until five years ago, when she woke up one morning and felt as if her entire body had fallen apart. She was fifty-eight years old. That was when she was finally diagnosed with fibromyalgia, but she believes she had this condition since she was a child. She has used her own experiences to help others, gathering and disseminating information on fibromyalgia to interested patients and medical professionals.

Sometimes we decide that knowing what we have isn't worth the trouble, particularly if little can be done to solve the problem. When a doctor first suggested that she had all the symptoms of fibromyalgia, Mireille, age fifty-one, wanted to know what could be done for her. Because her doctor said that fibromyalgia is a chronic condition she would have to learn to live with, Mireille decided, "It's not going to make much difference if I know for sure that's what I have." Yet she later discovered that having a definitive diagnosis helped her learn how to take care of herself. Exercise, medication to improve her sleep, and therapy have made a significant difference in Mireille's quality of life.

Disbelief from Others

We seek answers not only for ourselves but also to have something to tell our family, friends, and colleagues. Without a diagnosis, how can we expect them to believe we really are sick, especially when we question it so readily ourselves? It doesn't help that many of the illnesses we have are by and large invisible—pain and fatigue are hard to see.

When Jeri is not feeling well, she often gets the rash on her face that is characteristic of lupus. "I get nice rosy cheeks and I do look better," Jeri says. "I tell people I feel awful, and they say, 'You look wonderful.'" Kelly takes extra care to look good on days when she is feeling bad. "Often, times when I look the best, I feel the worst," she explains. As for me, because I'm self-employed, I can pad around my home office in sweats and no makeup, but sometimes I get depressed looking at myself in the mirror. Like Kelly, I may take extra care with my makeup or put on a favorite outfit to brighten my day. But I'm still tired, and I still hurt.

"If a person looks healthy, it is difficult to believe he or she may still be sick," Patricia Fennell points out. "If we do not see evidence of disease, we are suspicious and reach the conclusion that the person is lazy, malingering, or somehow immoral."[12]

I was troubled to find myself question my own son, who missed more than a month of ninth grade with chronic tonsillitis. There were days I thought he looked good enough to go to school. If I could suggest that he was not as sick as he said he was, knowing how much I hate it when someone disbelieves me, I began to understand how easy it must be for others to question how I feel. I also realized how helpless I felt in the face of my son's ongoing health problems and recognized my need to nudge him along the road to health.

Jeri tells me that before her diagnosis, there were times when her husband would ask her if she was lazy. "I vehemently said, 'No, I'm not lazy,'" Jeri says. "But when he added, 'You mean you're just going to sit in that chair today?' I said yes, because I was just that tired." At various times, I too have been told by people who love me that I am being "overly dramatic" or am "exaggerating my pain." In reality, I usually am exaggerating my health! Not wanting to be a burden to others or spoil their fun, I go along with planned activities no matter how I feel.

Self-Diagnosis

Because, like all people, we need some certainty around which to structure our lives, we are likely to come up with a diagnosis ourselves if we don't get one from our doctors. Pam, age thirty-nine, informed her doctor she had fibromyalgia eighteen months before he would confirm that diagnosis. She had been suffering with a number of related conditions for many years, including irritable bowel syndrome, a disorder marked by abdominal pain and intermittent constipation and diarrhea, which often accompanies fibromyalgia. "I thought it was normal," Pam says. "If I got sick when I ate cheesecake, I just didn't eat it anymore. It was my husband who pointed out that other people don't spend four hours a day in the bathroom."

Sometimes we get tired of running to the doctor with every new symptom. When pain in my arms was waking me up at night, and my hands went numb if I held them in certain positions, I confidently diagnosed myself with carpal tunnel syndrome. I was right about the diagnosis but wrong about the cause. I thought it was because as a writer and editor I type on a computer keyboard for long periods of time. By the time I was uncomfortable enough to visit my doctor, I learned I had developed a type of inflammatory arthritis that may accompany Sjogren's syndrome, and the swelling in my wrists was creating pressure on the median nerve that passes through the carpal tunnel into the palm of my hand. I wore cumbersome braces to sleep and to type, and I eventually required injection of anti-inflammatory medication in both wrists.

A Mixed Blessing

After years of self-blame and social stigma, a diagnosis may come as an enormous relief. We can stop trying either to deny or to prove that we are sick and can concentrate on getting better. Lexiann-Grant Snider, age thirty-nine, was "almost elated" to be diagnosed with Sjogren's syndrome. "Before," Lexiann says, "when I would really need to stop and rest, I would push through it and tell myself, 'You're not really sick.' Now I know I have a disease and I can go to bed and take care of myself." Lexiann's search for a diagnosis took her to twelve specialists. She began to fear she had something so rare that no one could help her, and she sank into a crippling depression that required hospitalization. Eventually, a doctor checking her for evidence of gallbladder disease discovered infiltration of lymphocytes in her gallbladder, liver, and pancreas. He diagnosed Lexiann with hepatitis and, subsequently, Sjogren's syndrome. In patients with Sjogren's syndrome, lymphocytes, a type of white blood cell that is supposed to protect the body by killing viruses and bacteria, invade and destroy body tissues instead. According to the Sjogren's Syndrome Foundation, autoimmune liver diseases commonly are found in association with Sjogren's syndrome.

For Jeri, the lupus diagnosis was confirmation that she is not depressed, lazy, or a hypochondriac. "Up to that point, I really felt mildly neurotic," Jeri says. Like Lexiann, Jeri's diagnosis also helped her begin to take care of herself. "Once you know what your disease is," she says, "you can find out what to do for yourself and what to expect." A definitive diagnosis was especially important for Linda Webb, who is adopted and has no way of knowing whether anyone in her birth family has inflammatory bowel disease. "I don't have a health history, so I don't know what to prevent," she says.

Even doctors seem to respond differently to us when our disease has a name. Author Linda Hanner reports that of 232 patients with chronic disease she surveyed, more than 60 percent said they were treated with more compassion by doctors after their illness was validated by a diagnosis.[13]

Unfortunately, our elation often is short-lived. Although a diagnosis initially may relieve stress, trauma specialist Patricia Fennell told me, "In reality, nothing has changed. You have a label, and, if you're really lucky, an acronym." If we had hoped a diagnosis would lead to a cure, we may be disappointed to learn that all we really can do is treat the symptoms. Further, the specific name we give our disease may have little to do with our treatment. I remember my rheumatologist patiently explaining to me that he was going to treat my arthritis the same way whether I had lupus, Sjogren's syndrome, or rheumatoid arthritis. I wanted a name to pin my hat on, but he was far more concerned with reducing the swelling in my joints, whatever the cause.

And those of us who hoped for some external validation may be dismayed to find that many people have never heard of our disease or don't believe it's real. Even some of the doctors I see are unaware of Sjogren's syndrome, and others believe that fibromyalgia is a manifestation of a psychological disorder. I often tell people I have something "like lupus," since Sjogren's and lupus are in the same family of autoimmune diseases. The names themselves reveal little. For example, Sjogren's syndrome is named for the Swedish ophthalmologist Henrik Sjögren, who wrote extensively about his clinical experience with patients who had dry eyes, dry mouth, and rheumatoid arthritis.

Our spouses also may be disheartened to learn that we can't readily be "fixed." Often, like us, they hope for a magic cure. Sally says her husband had an easier time when he believed she was just sick a lot. When she received a diagnosis of chronic fatigue syndrome while they were engaged, they had some serious discussions about whether he still wanted to marry her. We'll explore the impact of chronic illness on personal relationships in chapter 7.

PIECING THE PUZZLE TOGETHER

Even though a diagnosis may not yield the results we hope for, we go to great lengths to secure one. I have been poked, prodded, x-rayed, and scanned more times than I can count. In retrospect, I can see that my all-consuming search for answers was overshadowing my obvious need to take better care of myself. While I waited for someone else's permission to get better, I became sicker. My need for external validation was difficult to meet given the inexactness of medical science.

We don't like to be told that doctors don't know why we are sick. Yet there are any number of reasons why this might be the response we get. Whether we get a diagnosis and what specific diagnosis we get, may depend on the type of doctor we see, the particular symptoms we exhibit, the quality of the relationship we have with our doctors, and the reliability of the tests we are given.

Doctor Shopping

Perhaps one of the first lessons we learn in trying to pin a name on our disease is that our diagnosis is likely to depend on the type of doctor we see. "The patient who sees three doctors and receives three different diagnoses and treatment recommendations is beginning to learn something of the idiosyncratic nature of the diagnostic process," author Linda Hanner writes. "Thus the saying 'The doctor knows best' is ambiguous. It becomes a question of which doctor knows best."[14]

For her book *Healing Wounded Doctor–Patient Relationships,* Hanner surveyed 232 individuals with seven chronic illnesses (lupus, Lyme disease, multiple sclerosis, rheumatoid arthritis, fibromyalgia, interstitial cystitis, and myasthenia gravis) and discovered that the average length of time from onset of symptoms to diagnosis by a physician was at least two years.[15] The range across all illnesses was one month to forty-five years.[16]

The trend toward specialization in health care may be part of the problem. Two doctors can look at the same problem but name it in their own specialty. For example, a cardiologist may call pain in the chest wall costal chondritis, an inflammation of the cartilage between the ribs and the breastbone, while a rheumatologist may diagnose it as myofascial pain syndrome, a type of localized fibromyalgia. Treatment recommendations may differ depending on the diagnosis we receive. Specialization can be to our benefit, however, when the doctor we see is familiar with our problem.

By the time men and women find their way to the fibromyalgia treatment program at Oregon Health Sciences University (OHSU) in Portland, they have seen an average of eight physicians, according to professor of nursing Carol S. Burckhardt, a cofounder of the program. Most of her patients have been told there is nothing wrong or that they are suffering from depression, a diagnosis that may not square with their own understanding of their symptoms. "Finally they get to us and we say, 'This is what you have,' and they can stop that escalating quest to find an answer," she says.

For many of us, the search for answers takes us to far-flung places. Living in a small town in northwest Texas, Ken Henderson traveled to a hospital six hundred miles southeast of his home twice in two years to fig-ure out why he hurt so badly. He used vacation time from his job as head mechanic for the local school system. On his second visit, Ken was diag-nosed with fibromyalgia. Likewise, Lexiann Grant-Snider and her hus-band made numerous trips to out-of-town doctors before she was diagnosed with Sjogren's syndrome and hepatitis. There was little that doctors in her small southeastern Ohio town could do for her. The trips cost the Sniders financially as well as emotionally. Each time they saw a new doctor, they thought they had found an answer.

During our sometimes lengthy search to pin down a diagnosis, we may get a reputation for "doctor shopping." Those of us who see multiple doctors may be branded hypochondriacs or diagnosed with a psychiatric disorder. But often, all we are seeking is someone who believes that we are sick. When I finally found the rheumatologist who put the pieces of my medical puzzle together, I was a thirty-three-year-old single parent with a six-year-old son and a demanding new job. Having been told countless times that nothing was wrong with me, I told my new doctor I thought I was losing my mind. His response still brings tears to my eyes.

I believe you don't feel well. That's what my doctor said. It was a simple statement, honestly delivered, but it probably did more to relieve my mind and my physical suffering than anything anyone had done to that point. The self-recrimination that comes with being looked at as a hypochondriac or a malingerer can be as debilitating as any physical disease.

A Process of Exclusion

One of the problems in diagnosing chronic disease is that many ill-nesses share nonspecific or overlapping symptoms. Fatigue is a prime ex-ample of such a symptom. Though fatigue is one of the most common complaints patients have, according to Dr. Don Goldenberg, the subjective feeling of exhaustion that accompanies many chronic diseases is not mea-surable or well-defined.[17]

For ten years before I was diagnosed with Sjogren's syndrome and fi-bromyalgia, I felt as if I were looking out at the world through a thick fog. I wasn't tired just when I stayed up late, which I rarely had the energy to do, I was tired all the time. This was definitely not run-of-the-mill fatigue.

Like fatigue, pain is very individual and may be hard to define. Such adjectives as stabbing, throbbing, dull, burning, gnawing, and aching are used to describe pain, which results from stimulation of special sensory nerve endings because of injury or by disease.[18] We express and respond to pain differently based on our physiology, our prior experiences, and our culture's expectations. I remember a fellow participant in a stress management course for fibromyalgia patients saying to me, "You must be in a lot less pain than I am; I can't even function." But how could we compare our pain? Even if we had been able to measure it, perhaps we might have found that our pain was the same but we chose to respond to it differently. "All of us need to be careful not to pass judgment about the validity of someone else's pain," author Linda Hanner points out.[19]

Because fatigue, pain, and numerous other symptoms of chronic disease are vague or even overlapping, the diagnostic process often is one of exclusion; more serious illnesses must be ruled out first. "Certain illnesses are relatively easy to figure out," notes Dr. Richard A. Brown, a rheumatologist with Pioneer Health Center in Greenfield, Massachusetts. "With diabetes, you can measure blood sugar. Others, like chronic fatigue syndrome, fibromyalgia, and irritable bowel syndrome, are so nebulous they have to be determined by what you can see. There are no laboratory tests to prove or disprove that you have one of these illnesses." Lack of scientific proof of disease may be a major stumbling block in making a diagnosis. We'll take a further look at this problem later in this chapter.

Symptom Complexes

Even those diseases that include biological markers can be difficult to pin down because many of these illnesses are symptom complexes, and the symptoms don't come all at once. "With lupus, you may have joint pains one year and then you are tired another year and then maybe you have fevers," says Dr. Jill P. Buyon, associate professor of medicine at New York University School of Medicine. "It might be another two or three years before you actually get a rash on your face or become photosensitive."

Indeed, this was the case with my own diagnosis. Though early blood tests revealed that my body was making antibodies against itself, I had few of the major physical symptoms of either lupus or Sjogren's syndrome. Several years later, I developed inflammatory arthritis and learned that connective tissue diseases (those that are marked by inflammation in the muscles, joints, and skin) often accompany illnesses like Sjogren's. Together with my lab results and the clinical evidence of swollen salivary glands and arthritis, my doctor was willing to confirm a diagnosis of Sjogren's syndrome.

Kelly, who had been plagued for years by a series of seemingly un-connected symptoms including repeated episodes of hives, joint pain, and circulatory problems, unwittingly helped her doctor diagnosis lupus when she started visiting a tanning booth several years ago. Because ul-traviolet light can exacerbate lupus, Kelly became very ill after each tan-ning session. She was nauseous, stiff and achy, and extremely tired. "I was having individual symptoms for nearly ten years before finally I had mul-tiple symptoms at the same time," Kelly says. "If this hadn't happened, I could have gone for years with no diagnosis."

Sometimes our individual symptoms come and go so quickly, they are gone by the time we get to the doctor. I've always likened this phe-nomenon to taking your car to the mechanic only to have it not squeak when you get there. Jeri recalls, "I'd have this really raging sore in my mouth, make an appointment to see the dentist, and before I could get there the sore would be gone."

Likewise, though I never knew precisely when my glands would be swollen, I knew they wouldn't be when I got to the doctor's office. Finally, I started asking doctors if I could make a same-day appointment the next time I woke up looking like a chipmunk. I made one appointment to dis-cuss my concerns and another to show the physical evidence to three dif-ferent doctors—a primary care physician, an otolaryngologist (ears, nose, and throat specialist), and a rheumatologist, each of whom referred me to the next specialist. I was getting tired of disrupting my life to run to doc-tors, but my persistence paid off. The final physician I saw—the rheuma-tologist—was the one who eventually diagnosed me with both Sjogren's syndrome and fibromyalgia. Often, we must rally to be our own best ad-vocate when we feel least able to do so.

Doctor–Patient Communication

When we've made the medical rounds for months or even years, we may begin to feel that our disease is hard to diagnose. In part, this may be the result of poor doctor–patient communication, according to Dr. Jill Buyon. "Doctors say things like, 'We don't know what you have,' but maybe they really don't mean it that way," she says. "They may mean it can't be categorized at the moment, and then the frustrated patient thinks it's hard to diagnose the disease."

She offers an example. "Say a woman has very bad joint complaints and a positive lupus test. Well, those are only two abnormalities. Do I tell her I don't know what she has? Do I tell her she is prelupus? I happen to tell her that she has an undifferentiated autoimmune disease, but she may interpret that to mean that I don't know what she has. I *do* know what she has," Dr. Buyon notes, "but what I don't have is a crystal ball to tell whether or not she will meet criteria for lupus in the future."

We may also be victims of our own expectations. "Many patients push to have a diagnosis, but a doctor can't be forced to give a name to something the patient doesn't have," Dr. Buyon says. Both patients and doctors expect the doctor to come up with a diagnosis, and when one is not forthcoming, "blame is often assigned to the doctor for being incompetent or to the patient for imagining or feigning symptoms," author Linda Hanner writes.[20] I know that each time a doctor handed me a clean bill of health, I vacillated between thinking either I was crazy or the doctor was missing something important. The doctor–patient relationship is examined in more detail in chapter 3.

Diagnostic Tests

When my rheumatologist told me that my blood test results indicated lupus, though I lacked any observable symptoms of the disease, I quickly learned one of the paradoxes of making a medical diagnosis: we can have "positive" medical tests in the absence of observable clinical symptoms, and we can have physical manifestations of illness without any corroborating laboratory results. For example, patients with rheumatoid arthritis may show no evidence of specific antibodies called a rheumatoid factor and, conversely, people with a positive rheumatoid factor may never develop arthritis. Our doctors, therefore, must rely both on what they observe and what our laboratory tests reveal. However, many patients and doctors alike are concerned about the medical profession's increasing reliance on technology, a topic we'll explore in more depth in chapter 3. "In the old days, doctors diagnosed people by observing them and listening to their complaints," says Cindy Perlin, a clinical social worker in private practice in Delmar, New York. "Now, doctors send you for tests. If the tests don't show anything, you're not sick."

The problem with many medical tests is that the results may be inconclusive and, even when certain, may have little impact on our treatment. My rheumatologist talked me out of having a lip biopsy, a test used to confirm the presence of lymphocytic infiltration common in Sjogren's syndrome. He told me the procedure itself was painful and that, regardless of what the test revealed, he would continue treating me for Sjogren's syndrome based on the bulk of evidence he had collected already. I'm grateful to this day for my doctor's advice; I've talked to a number of people who have had inconclusive results from this test and who have been left with a lingering numbness in their lip.

An equivocal medical test can be emotionally devastating. When he suspected Sjogren's syndrome, Kathy Hammitt's doctor sent her to the University of Virginia in Charlottesville for further testing. She was home alone with her infant daughter when a resident from the hospital called to tell her that she had lymphoma, a cancer of the lymph glands that develops in fewer than 5 percent of Sjogren's patients. The resident said it would take three months to schedule a CAT scan to confirm the diagnosis. Computerized axial tomography (CAT), or whole body scanning, is a diagnostic technique that combines the use of a computer and X rays to produce clear, cross-sectional images of the tissue being examined.

"I told him that was too long to wait, but he said it wasn't going to make a difference in the prognosis anyway," Kathy says. She scheduled a CAT scan at a local hospital and was prepared to have a swollen thymus gland (part of the body's immune system) removed, when a doctor suggested that she adopt a wait-and-see attitude. Kathy did not develop lymphoma, but she has since had a second false scare. "You would like to think you've found a way to cope with a potentially life-threatening situation, but it doesn't get any easier to go through," she says.

Uncertain tests leave us in a state of limbo. Though she had symptoms of Lyme disease, Joan O'Brien-Singer, age fifty-seven, was told repeatedly that the results of blood tests that could confirm the diagnosis were equivocal. She was reluctant to start treatment until she had a definitive answer. Eventually, someone gave her the name of an internist who treats patients with Lyme disease, and he told Joan that "'equivocal' is like being 'a little bit pregnant.'" He diagnosed her with Lyme disease, which is an infectious, tick-transmitted disorder that results in flu-like symptoms and joint inflammation. According to the Centers for Disease Control, a record 16,461 cases of Lyme disease were reported in the United States in 1996, a 41 percent increase over 1995. The agency attributes the increase to changes in the tick population, greater awareness of Lyme disease, and better reporting.[21]

First identified in Old Lyme, Connecticut, in 1975, Lyme disease is especially prevalent in the New England and mid-Atlantic states, where new cases increased by 99 percent between 1995 and 1996. Lyme disease is the most common tick-borne infection in Europe, though prevalence rates are hard to determine because of varying surveillance methods, according to the European Union for Concerted Action on Lyme Borreliosis.[22] In its early stages, Lyme disease can be treated successfully with antibiotics. There is ongoing disagreement in the medical and scientific communities about the existence of a chronic condition linked to Lyme disease. Some doctors, like Dr. Don Goldenberg, believe that individuals with chronic Lyme disease actually have fibromyalgia or chronic fatigue syndrome precipitated by the Lyme infection.[23]

In addition to being inconclusive, medical tests for chronic disease may be painful and, depending on our financial resources, prohibitively expensive. To confirm a diagnosis of interstitial cystitis, Lois Arias, age forty-five, had her bladder filled and distended with water to check for pinpoint hemorrhages on the bladder wall that are indicative of this disease. This procedure is termed a hydrodistension and is typically done under general anesthesia. I also have been diagnosed with interstitial cystitis, and I was in considerable pain the first time I tried to urinate after having the hydrodistension. My fiancé accompanied me to the same-day procedure, and I was frightened to be alone when he had to return home that evening. Lois, however, had a particularly bad reaction. "I had to use a catheter for a week because I couldn't urinate on my own," Lois says. "It took me two months to get back to the pain level I had before the procedure." To help others dealing with this condition, Lois became coleader of an interstitial cystitis support group on America Online. Discussion of the Internet as a resource for information and support is featured in chapter 6.

Lenore, age forty-four, started having frequent urinary tract infections in her late twenties. When her symptoms could no longer be controlled by antibiotics, her urologist suggested she might have interstitial cystitis. With no health insurance, Lenore couldn't afford the $3,000 out-of-pocket expense for the hydrodistension her doctor recommended. "Financially, it was going to be too much for me to get that diagnosis," Lenore says, "so I just thought, 'Well, if I have it, I have it.'" Though there are numerous treatments for interstitial cystitis, there is no known cause or cure.

DISEASES AND SYNDROMES

The medical problems we've discussed thus far fall into two categories—diseases and syndromes. Diseases such as multiple sclerosis and lupus are marked by measurable, physiological abnormalities. A syndrome like fibromyalgia or chronic fatigue syndrome is characterized by a collection of symptoms we report to the doctor and physical signs that he or she can see. Syndromes may cause us to be ill in the absence of any observable disease. The lack of laboratory results to confirm many syndromes may hinder the diagnostic process.

The American College of Rheumatology issued diagnostic criteria for fibromyalgia in 1990. Patients must have widespread pain in all four quadrants of the body for a minimum of three months and at least eleven of eighteen specified tender points. In 1994, the Centers for Disease Control issued guidelines for a diagnosis of chronic fatigue syndrome. They include severe, unexplained fatigue that lasts for six or more consecutive months and is not relieved by rest, along with at least four of eight additional symptoms such as sore throat, muscle pain, and impaired memory or concentration problems.[24]

But even though there are objective diagnostic criteria, with very few laboratory data to support a pathologic process, many doctors are reluctant to consider fibromyalgia and chronic fatigue syndrome as legitimate diseases. "There are some physicians who will refuse to believe that fibromyalgia and chronic fatigue syndrome are real entities until there is a blood test you can draw that will be abnormal in most people with these illnesses and normal in most people who don't have them," says Dr. Daniel J. Clauw, assistant professor of medicine at Georgetown University Medical Center. Because he believes these illnesses may reflect abnormalities of the central nervous system that will be difficult to measure, Dr. Clauw adds, "I'm not sure that's ever going to happen."

Some physicians fear that giving patients a diagnosis of fibromyalgia or chronic fatigue syndrome encourages them to think of themselves as ill, according to Dr. Don Goldenberg. However, most of us who are sick view a diagnosis as important information that points us in the direction of getting better. Because such illnesses are more common in women, Dr. Goldenberg suggests that "gender bias" may play a role in this debate. He writes that the prevalence of fibromyalgia and chronic fatigue syndrome in women confirms the belief some doctors hold that women tend to react psychosomatically, more so than men, when life is hard. "It could more cogently be argued that such illness is related to hormonal factors in women. It may even be related to the stress of living in a male-dominated society where female problems are brushed aside."[25] Because I was working full-time and caring for a small child, none of the physicians I saw seemed to intimate that I was a "bored housewife," as some women have been told. Nor did I find that male physicians were necessarily dismissive. However, I did feel that some doctors, both male and female, were less willing or able than others to respond to my concerns. We'll talk more about the role of a doctor's knowledge and beliefs in chapter 3.

Overlapping Syndromes

Many doctors who treat patients with fibromyalgia and chronic fatigue syndrome believe these illnesses are two sides of the same coin, with pain being the predominant feature of fibromyalgia and debilitating fatigue the cardinal symptom of chronic fatigue syndrome. Recent research suggests that other chronic disorders also may be related to one another. For example, Dr. Muhammad B. Yunus, professor of medicine at the University of Illinois College of Medicine at Peoria, believes that fibromyalgia is part of what he calls dysregulation spectrum syndrome, or DSS, which also includes such illnesses as chronic fatigue syndrome, irritable bowel syndrome, and migraine headaches, among others.[26] The concept of DSS, according to Dr. Yunus, is based on the fact that these types of illnesses tend to cluster in the same individuals, share many symptoms, respond to a similar group of medications, and are likely to result from abnormalities in the body's neurological, hormonal, and immune system functions.

In particular, individuals with fibromyalgia have been shown to have several times the normal amount of substance P, a peripheral pain neurotransmitter, in their spinal fluid.[27] At the same time, serum levels of serotonin—a neurotransmitter that controls sleep states, consciousness, and moods—and its precursor, the essential amino acid tryptophan, are low in these people. Neurotransmitters are chemical messengers that transmit nerve impulses in the body. Under normal circumstances, substance P would initiate a pain signal following injury, and serotonin would reduce the intensity of that signal.[28] These abnormalities might help explain the pain and fatigue that constitute fibromyalgia.

Though a precise cause of such illnesses as fibromyalgia and chronic fatigue syndrome has not been determined, a growing body of research points to a dysregulation of the autonomic nervous system. We'll explore some of these studies in more detail in chapter 2. The autonomic nervous system, made up of the sympathetic and the parasympathetic branches, is that part of the nervous system that controls involuntary or automatic functions, such as heart rate and breathing. The sympathetic nervous system prepares the body for action by activating the so-called fight-or-flight response that allows us to react to internal or external stressors. Patients with fibromyalgia and related conditions may have an impaired ability to respond to stress that indicates exhaustion of the autonomic system from chronic stimulation, according to Dr. Daniel Clauw.[29]

This line of inquiry squares with my own experience of fibromyalgia. Many days I feel as if my insides are moving while the rest of me is standing still; I am seemingly overstimulated and exhausted at the same time. As tired as I might be, I often have to keep moving to balance the internal and external sensations I experience.

Like fibromyalgia, chronic fatigue syndrome, and chronic Lyme disease, Gulf War syndrome often is dismissed as a "wastebasket" diagnosis, one that encompasses a number of problems that may not represent disease. There is little consensus within the federal government or the scientific and medical communities about the possible causes of veterans' complaints of fatigue, joint pain, memory loss, and stomach disorders. Everything from exposure to toxic chemicals to the stress of war has been blamed, but no definitive conclusions have been drawn. In October 1996, a panel of the National Academy of Science's Institute of Medicine said it preferred the term *unexplained illness* to Gulf War syndrome.[30]

Appearing before the U.S. Congress in March 1996, Dr. Clauw, who has received several federal research grants to study illnesses associated with service in the Persian Gulf, testified that Gulf War syndrome is part of the broad spectrum of health disorders that includes fibromyalgia and chronic fatigue syndrome.[31] He believes that individuals may inherit a predisposition for this type of central nervous system dysfunction and that the illness itself is triggered by a physical, immune system, or emotional stressor. "Individuals deployed to the Persian Gulf may have been exposed to any or all of these stressors," he said. We'll take a more detailed look at the relationship between stress and chronic illness in chapter 2.

Depression and Chronic Disease

DSS and similar models are predominantly biomedical. Other researchers consider these disorders to be part of a spectrum of psychiatric conditions, in part because of a perceived prevalence of depression among people with such illnesses as fibromyalgia and irritable bowel syndrome. Though a minority of people with fibromyalgia have a psychological problem, even after controlling for the effect of chronic disease Dr. Muhammad Yunus and others have concluded that fibromyalgia and depression are biologically different conditions.[32] In fact, in Dr. Yunus's earlier work, including the article cited in this chapter, he called DSS *dysfunctional* spectrum syndrome, but more recently has begun using the term *dysregulation* because he believes that *dysfunctional* wrongly implies that these illnesses are psychiatric in origin.[33] In many cases, individuals may develop mood disorders such as depression or anxiety *as a result* of their physical symptoms. Indeed, a number of doctors suggested that I was sick because I was depressed, but I thought I was depressed because I was sick. The intricate relationship between depression and other chronic illnesses is examined in chapter 2.

Co-occurring Syndromes and Diseases

In many cases, a syndrome such as fibromyalgia may coexist with an autoimmune disease. Drs. Daniel Clauw and Paul Katz estimate that one third of individuals with autoimmune disorders have concurrent fibromyalgia, which is considerably higher than the percentage of people who have fibromyalgia in the general population (approximately 2 to 4 percent).[34] A causal relationship between fibromyalgia and rheumatic disorders has not been determined, but doctors do know that the overlap of these conditions may intensify the symptoms of both illnesses. In addition, the symptoms of these co-occurring disorders become intertwined, and it can be difficult to pull them apart. When I'm tired and I hurt all over, I sometimes wonder which illness is to blame, but this can be a pointless exercise. On bad days, it's more useful for me to accept the fact that I don't feel well, period, and take the steps I need to feel better.

MOVING FORWARD

The first months and years we are sick are marked by fear, uncertainty, and denial. We wearily make the rounds of doctors, who may or may not be able to diagnose our condition. Understandably, we feel a desperate need to know why we are sick so we can understand how to get better. Feeling better is always the bottom line. But, ironically, our tireless pursuit of a diagnosis may keep us from taking care of ourselves. Looking back, I can see that I could have rested when I was tired, said no when I was overcommitted, and asked for help at work and at home even before my health problems were named. My need to be certain kept me stuck in illness when I could have been moving forward to better health.

And what about the outside validation we seek? That may need to come from within. Dr. Ernesto Vasquez, a psychiatrist in private practice in Columbus, Ohio, has been diagnosed with both fibromyalgia and chronic fatigue syndrome. When I asked him how he felt about having not one but two illnesses that many of his colleagues don't believe in, he replied, "It requires that I be credible with myself." This is a critical lesson for a successful life, with or without chronic disease, and one that I am still working hard to learn.

Throughout this book, we'll examine how those of us with chronic illnesses strike a delicate balance between understanding our illnesses and learning to live with them. Being sick every day is a life-altering event, and how we respond to this unexpected change teaches us much about ourselves.

A STUMBLING BLOCK

Is My Illness Really "All in My Head"?

It is arrogant of us as scientists to feel that because we cannot
precisely define a problem, it doesn't exist.[1]
DR. DANIEL J. CLAUW

The original working title of this book was *It's Not All in Your Head*. I
chose that because many of us have struggled with some significant
questions. Are we physically ill or are we depressed? Is our illness caused
by stress? Most important, are we to blame for being sick? The answers to
these questions are at once complex and reassuring, and we'll explore
them in this chapter. In particular, we'll look at changing thoughts about
the interrelationship of the mind and the body in the production of disease. We'll explore the connection between depression and other chronic
illnesses, and examine the role of stress in our disease. Also, we'll touch
on the cognitive problems that often accompany many chronic illnesses.
Finally, we'll discuss the notion of blame. Even if we are depressed or
under a great deal of stress, we are not at fault for being sick. We are,
however, responsible for getting well.

SORTING OUT THE MIND AND THE BODY

I grew up thinking that my emotions affected my body. When I was a small child, my mother told me that if I pouted my face would freeze in that position. When I was in my early twenties, my family doctor suggested that I must be depressed because I was having frequent urinary tract and vaginal infections. When friends learned I had arthritis, they offered the conventional wisdom that arthritis is anger turned inward. I struggled with this notion because I thought I was being told that if I were happier, my physical symptoms would go away. When I still felt ill at otherwise joyous moments in my life, I became frustrated and confused.

Hippocrates and Descartes

To understand more about the relationship of the mind (psyche) and the body (soma), and how we can use this knowledge, we have to examine a bit of history. Hippocrates, a Greek physician of the fourth century B.C. who is widely credited as being the father of medicine, believed in a delicate interrelationship between the mind and the body. He maintained that a person's physical symptoms were affected by his or her psychological state, spiritual leanings, and social connections.[2] Hippocrates's works were lost during the Middle Ages but were rediscovered during the Renaissance when Western physicians had direct access to Greek scholars and texts.

This integrated view of mind and body began to shift during the early seventeenth century, however, when some prominent European philosophers, such as England's Francis Bacon and France's René Descartes, were beginning to develop the worldview that underlies today's Western medicine. "Some of the great Renaissance physicians still believed, as Hippocrates did, that matter and spirit were connected," says Dr. James S. Gordon, director of the Center for Mind–Body Medicine in Washington, D.C. "So far as Descartes was concerned, however, there was a definitive separation between the mind and the body."[3]

This Cartesian split between the mind and the body informs today's biomedical model of medicine, in which doctors seek physical causes for disease. Those illnesses that don't result in measurable physiological abnormalities may be discredited or discounted.

"Those things that are physical, concrete, measurable, observable, and quantifiable are considered organic and elevated to the status of 'real,'" says clinical social worker and trauma specialist Patricia Fennell, president of Albany Health Management Associates. "We assign what can't be measured to the psychological and discount it." We may even blame people who have an illness we don't understand. For example, Fennell points out, the term *yuppie flu* is a derogatory description for chronic fatigue syndrome, whose sufferers are believed to be successful, white, middle-class women who "were greedily trying to have it all and, as a result, got just what they deserved."[4] In actuality, according to a recent University of Washington study, "chronic fatigue looks the same, feels the same, and appears with the same frequency in nonwhites as in whites."[5] Researchers found no overall differences between white and nonwhite participants in age, sex, level of education, or reported symptoms of chronic fatigue syndrome.

New Age Thinking

More recently, with the help of so-called New Age philosophers and proponents of non-Western medical practices, the winds have begun to shift again. Today, the much-touted connection between mind and body is the subject of numerous best-selling books, television specials, and self-help tapes. But the pendulum may have swung too far in the other direction. Now, instead of being told that if no physical cause for our illness can be found it must be "all in our heads," we learn that what's in our heads might be making us sick. "Today's New Age thinking promotes the assumption that if you live the examined life, you should be well," Patricia Fennell told me. The idea is that if we have had enough therapy, done enough introspection, and examined our spiritual beliefs, we will uncover the reasons why we "need" to be sick and will be able to make ourselves well. There is, indeed, a complex interplay between mood and health, as we'll see throughout this chapter, but taken to the extreme this attitude becomes a not-so-subtle way to blame the victim of chronic disease. Since I couldn't seem to "think myself well" despite having done all of the requisite self-examination, I began to feel that my mind was as defective as my body, and I ended up feeling worse.

Examining the "Mindbody"

The truth of the matter is, the mind–body issue is enormously complex. "It is impossible to separate the mind from the body," Linda Hanner writes in *Healing Wounded Doctor–Patient Relationships.* "Diseases that disrupt the body's hormonal or chemical balance can present themselves as psychiatric disorders, and psychiatric disorders can be accompanied by very real physical symptoms."[6]

The intricate relationship between the human mind and body lead many to believe they are inseparable. While researching this book, I took a six-week course for people with chronic illness sponsored by my health plan. The aim of the course was to improve participants' mood and health, and presumably to cut back on our need for more expensive medical care. In the course, we talked about the *mindbody*—one word, no hyphen.

In her clinical practice working with people who have chronic diseases, Patricia Fennell says she always assumes a physical corollary to psychological problems, and vice versa. "Mind–body is a false dichotomy," she says. Professor of nursing Carol S. Burckhardt, a cofounder of the OHSU fibromyalgia treatment program, agrees. "You have to get people out of the mind–body dichotomy. Once you do, to say that somebody's muscular pain is a manifestation of depression doesn't even make sense," she says.

Labels

Why do we and our doctors sometimes struggle with the need to find a purely physical or a purely psychological cause for our disease? "The desire to put labels on everything leads us to divide illnesses into two main categories—the psychogenic and the organic (physical)," author Linda Hanner says. "As a result, many doctors are quick to throw the problems of those who don't have clearly defined physical ailments into the psychological wastebasket."[7] As we saw in chapter 1, many doctors refuse to believe there is a physical cause for illnesses that have no easily identifiable biological markers. This may have to do in part with those doctors' sense of competence. "Some doctors turn away patients with fibromyalgia or chronic fatigue syndrome because they are frustrated at their inability to treat them," says Dr. Daniel J. Clauw, assistant professor of medicine at Georgetown University Medical Center. "Our job is to help, and we feel helpless in the face of these diseases. Some doctors push patients away overtly, by saying they can't help, or subliminally, by telling them their problems are all in their head."

For our part, we may fear to be labeled a hypochondriac or, worse, mentally ill. I have been writing about mental illness for nearly ten years, and I am well aware that most serious psychiatric disorders, including depression, are considered to be diseases of the brain, just as diabetes is a disorder of the pancreas. Still, stigma is hard to overcome, and I felt that even my doctors might take my complaints more seriously if they thought they were dealing with a "real" disease. I wanted and needed to believe that I was depressed because I was sick and not sick because I was depressed. In terms of treatment, I came to realize it probably was a moot point, as we'll discover in the following pages. But in terms of how I feel about myself and how others see me, I still have a difficult time accepting the fact that, for me, mild depression is inextricably intertwined with my physical health.

DEPRESSION AND CHRONIC DISEASE

If we haven't been told outright that our problems are all in our head, we frequently have had doctors suggest that we may be experiencing psychological problems. "What may begin as a suspicion of a psychological disorder for the physician or a somatization disorder (bodily complaints for which no physical cause can be found) for the behavioral health care provider may become an allegation of deliberate malingering," Patricia Fennell writes.[8] Our emotions may indeed play a critical role in shaping our physical health, but we still have bodily symptoms that need our doctors' attention.

A number of the people I interviewed told me that at some point in their search for a diagnosis, at least one doctor they saw intimated that their physical health problems were caused by psychological factors—everything from wanting to avoid school to marital problems to sibling rivalry. When my family doctor suggested that chronic vaginal and urinary tract infections had left me feeling depressed, he seemed equally concerned about my husband. He suggested that because my husband had been deprived of my affections, the marriage might be troubled, and that *that* could be affecting my mood. Actually, I was just tired of being in pain and on antibiotics!

Few of us have had an experience as dramatic as Ken Henderson's, however. His doctor suggested he see another physician in a neighboring town. "I thought I was just going to see another doctor for the pain I was having," recalls Ken, who later was diagnosed with fibromyalgia. "When I got to the hospital, there were two nurses waiting outside. They escorted me upstairs through double doors that read *Mental Ward* and proceeded to show me how to get the toilet paper off the dispenser and how to flush the commode. Then they took me down to another room where I would be in basket-weaving classes. I told them I was in the wrong place, and I checked myself out. I didn't want to weave baskets." Ken's doctor apologized for the misunderstanding; he only intended for Ken to discover whether anxiety might be making his physical condition worse.

Mireille, who also has fibromyalgia, said no to a doctor for the first time in her life when he wanted her to continue taking antidepressant medication despite debilitating side effects. "He seemed to be quite concerned about the fact that I was depressed, while I thought I was taking the antidepressant to help me with my fibromyalgia." Low doses of various antidepressant medications frequently are used to treat the sleep and mood disorders associated with fibromyalgia and related illnesses. "I realized we weren't on the same wavelength at all," she adds. "My doctor was treating a depressed woman in premenopause, and I was looking for somebody to treat my fibromyalgia. Those are two different things."

Similar but Not the Same

Dr. Daniel Clauw agrees that although depression and fibromyalgia may co-occur, they are distinct illnesses. "Fibromyalgia is primarily a physical illness," Dr. Clauw told me. He notes that studies that have examined the overlap between psychiatric illnesses and fibromyalgia find that about 30 to 40 percent of patients with fibromyalgia or chronic fatigue syndrome have some sort of concurrent psychiatric problem. "What this means," he explains, "is that 60 percent to 70 percent of people with fibromyalgia or chronic fatigue syndrome have no identifiable psychiatric problem at all. Obviously, in that group of people, there have to be very organic, physiological reasons for their pain and fatigue."

Patients with fibromyalgia do, however, have a higher incidence of psychiatric disorders than the general population. For example, in large community samples, only approximately 4 percent of individuals have diagnosable depression.[9] Because of this discrepancy, Dr. Clauw writes,

> Considerable controversy surrounds the relationship between these psychiatric conditions and the concurrent physical symptoms. Some believe that fibromyalgia is primarily a psychiatric condition and that the related symptoms are the result of somatization, whereas others believe that psychiatric problems largely occur as a consequence of the chronic pain, fatigue, and disability these patients have. This de-

bate becomes less relevant if the psychiatric disturbances are considered in the same light as physical symptoms in that there is a common neurotransmitter or hormonal imbalance responsible, and thus both occur in increased frequency in patients with fibromyalgia.[10]

Depression also may accompany autoimmune diseases such as Sjogren's syndrome and lupus. "Each of the autoimmune disorders has been associated with mood, behavioral, and cognitive changes," write Drs. Susan Swedo and Henrietta Leonard, two of the nation's top mental health experts. "Depression is fairly common and may be the result of inflammation of blood vessels within the brain."[11]

The distinction between depression and chronic illness becomes blurred when we have clinical depression coexisting with another disease. To escape a violent marriage, Dulce shot herself. It was the mid-1950s, and she felt she had few other options. "It was the law that if you survived, you must have psychiatric help," she says. "With that on my record, no matter what I saw a doctor for after that, I was told I was depressed or that my problems were all in my head." Looking back, Dulce firmly believes that in most cases, her fibromyalgia was causing her depression rather than the other way around. A fibromyalgia flare landed her in a psychiatric hospital in the mid-1970s, but Dulce feels lucky because her psychiatrist prescribed antidepressant medication that helped her fibromyalgia symptoms.

Wendy Hay, age thirty-four, has been treated for clinical depression since the age of twenty. In March 1996, she was diagnosed with multiple sclerosis. Before she received her newest diagnosis, Wendy began experiencing cognitive difficulties similar to depressive symptoms even though she was taking her antidepressant medication. At first, she ignored the early warning signs of a change in her health and attributed them to her depression.

Depression and Loss

Even if we don't have a diagnosable mental illness, there are any number of reasons why being sick might cause us to feel depressed. In her work with fibromyalgia patients at Oregon Health Sciences University, nurse Carol Burckhardt says, "Many people find they've given up most of the pleasurable things in life and they're focusing on getting dressed, going to work, and feeding the family. No wonder they're depressed." Because there is a higher prevalence of depression in people with fibromyalgia, the staff screens individuals carefully, but Burckhardt adds, "Everybody who has a chronic illness where there is a lot of uncertainty has depressive symptoms."

For many of us with chronic disease, fear of the future is one of the most difficult problems we face. When I learned I had arthritis, I was relieved to know that my pain was real but I was devastated at the thought that I faced an uncertain future. At that point I didn't know that the type of inflammatory arthritis that accompanies Sjogren's syndrome typically is not disabling. Visions of being in a wheelchair haunted me; I had a young child to care for.

In addition to fearing the future, people with chronic diseases face any numbers of losses, notes social worker Cindy Perlin of Delmar, New York. "Even if you're leading a perfectly happy, healthy, well-rounded life and you're coping well, once you become ill, that brings a whole new set of problems," Perlin says. Often we lose friends, income, and, worst of all, our own sense of self-esteem. The emotional impact of ongoing illness is discussed in more detail in chapter 6.

Being sick and not being believed can make us a bit "neurotic," author Linda Hanner suggests. "Few physicians realize the torment people go through when they are being told or are trying to convince themselves they should be able to function normally, but they can't."[12] As I noted earlier, I still get teary-eyed when I think about the rheumatologist who first said, *I believe you don't feel well*. None of us wants to be thought of as a hypochondriac or a malingerer, and our fear that we might be imagining our symptoms makes our physical condition worse. Indeed, so many of us struggle with self-blame that I have devoted special attention to this topic later in the chapter.

Motivated Patients

Some doctors say they can tell fairly easily whether they're dealing with a person who is depressed. "Usually the doctor has a real sense of when there is psychopathology," says Dr. Richard A. Brown, a rheumatologist with Pioneer Health Center in Greenfield, Massachusetts. "It's not subtle. When we see a well-intentioned, fairly high-functioning individual who comes in with lots of complaints, we take them seriously." Dr. Brown further notes, "If I can tell that the patient is trying to get better and not just sitting in my office saying, 'Okay, doctor make me well,' that's a tip-off."

Dr. Paul Cheney, a North Carolina physician noted for his research in chronic fatigue syndrome, found that while people who are depressed often lose interest in everything, patients with chronic fatigue syndrome are just the opposite. He told *Newsweek* magazine, "'They're terribly concerned about what their symptoms mean. They can't function. They can't work. Many are petrified. But they do not lack interest in their surroundings.'"[13]

Pam expresses this distinction with a liberal dose of humor. Told for years before her fibromyalgia diagnosis that her symptoms were all in her head, Pam says, "It was very frustrating for me because I figured if I were going to lose my mind, I probably would have a lot more fun. I wouldn't even care at that point. But I cared very much about how I felt."

The Complex Interplay of Mood and Health

If we become defensive when a doctor suggests that our illness might have a psychological basis, Linda Hanner believes it only causes the doctor to become more suspicious that our illness may be a psychiatric problem.[4] Exploring the role of emotional difficulties in physical illness can be important, Hanner believes, and the doctor who validates a patient's physical symptoms leaves the door open to exploring psychological factors.

Indeed, when I complained of fatigue to my family doctor, and he gave me a prescription for a strong antidepressant without suggesting I talk to anyone about what might be bothering me, I threw the medication away. But had my doctor taken the time to acknowledge that I wasn't feeling well physically and to explain the relationship between emotional and physical health, I might have been more willing to follow his suggestions. In retrospect, his advice might have been on the mark, given what I now know about the role of antidepressant medication in treating such illnesses as fibromyalgia. But I rejected his recommendation because I thought he hadn't taken my concerns seriously.

"When you're consulting with a reliable physician about some of your symptoms, and you get an answer that you feel doesn't address the issue, you just decide this person cannot hear what you're saying," Jeri says. Some of us reject out of hand our doctor's suggestion that we get psychological help. Others follow through only to get confirmation that they are not depressed. Ken Henderson spent four months with a psychiatrist the year before he was diagnosed with fibromyalgia. "The doctor said that as far as he was concerned, I was as normal as he was," Ken laughs. "He thought I got depressed occasionally because everybody was telling me that nothing was wrong." Still others among us find that psychological counseling or self-help groups can be a lifeline for dealing with chronic disease, a topic we'll explore in more detail in chapter 6.

Ironically, when I finally decided that I wanted to try antidepressants to ease my fibromyalgia symptoms, I was referred to a psychiatrist who said he could find no evidence that I was depressed! He probed for the classic signs of clinical depression, such as lack of interest in activities I previously enjoyed. I told him I was still keeping up with my life, I was just tired and achy while I was doing it. However, he was willing to let me try medication for premenstrual mood swings that left me feeling drained and ashamed that I could be so grouchy. Many women with chronic illness find that the symptoms of their disease become worse just before their period. So in a roundabout way I received the help I needed, but it still makes me laugh to think that years ago, a general practitioner suggested I was depressed while, more recently, a psychiatrist said that I wasn't. The complex interplay between mood and health makes many chronic illnesses difficult to diagnose and treat.

COGNITIVE PROBLEMS

Cognitive changes are particularly troubling for many of us with chronic disease and may lead to increased concern about the state of our mental health. We may think one word but say another, substitute a description for a common word we can't remember, transpose numbers and letters in speech and writing, draw a complete blank in the middle of a thought, or forget our telephone number or our wedding anniversary. As Katrina Berne notes in an article appropriately titled, "Life on Seven Brain Cells a Day," cognitive problems are "especially difficult for those who have relied heavily on their intellectual abilities and who have derived meaning and pleasure from their ability to think clearly and well."[15] As for me, I have always taken great pride in my intelligence, possibly to the detriment of my emotional health. Now, I have no choice but to develop further my "softer side" because many days, my once sharp-as-a-tack brain feels like oatmeal.

A Common Phenomenon

You won't hear too many people with chronic illness talk about cognitive problems because we are afraid of being perceived as incapable of meeting our responsibilities. Yet this is a fairly common symptom of many diseases. Cognitive dysfunction, including memory loss, forgetfulness, poor concentration, and confusion, may affect as many as two thirds of fibromyalgia patients.[16] Impaired memory or concentration problems is one of the Centers for Disease Control's diagnostic criteria for chronic fatigue syndrome.

The neurocognitive disturbances experienced by people with such illnesses as fibromyalgia and chronic fatigue syndrome are similar to those seen in people recovering from head trauma or injuries, according to Dr. Don L. Goldenberg, chief of rheumatology and director of the Arthritis/ Fibromyalgia Center at Newton-Wellesley Hospital in Newton, Massachusetts. He believes that in people with these syndromes, the cognitive symptoms may result from decreased blood flow to the brain.[17] There is, however, no evidence of significant brain injury or inflammation. Multiple factors may contribute to cognitive dysfunction, including mood disorders, medications, fatigue, pain, and sleep disturbances.

Individuals with certain autoimmune diseases show evidence of cognitive impairment too. In a study of individuals with lupus, researchers reported that 80 percent of participants with neuropsychiatric involvement (such as headaches, seizures, and psychosis) and 42 percent of participants who never had neuropsychiatric symptoms demonstrated significant cognitive impairment. This compares with 17 percent of patients with rheumatoid arthritis and 14 percent of controls. The cause of central nervous system involvement in lupus is not well understood at this time, and may include multiple mechanisms.[18]

Brain Fog

Those of us with such illnesses as fibromyalgia and chronic fatigue syndrome refer to this phenomenon as *brain fog*. I have often thought that the movie *Joe Versus the Volcano*, in which Tom Hanks plays a man plagued by a "rare" condition his physician calls a "brain cloud," should be required viewing for everyone with chronic disease (though I doubt many of us would jump into a volcano to relieve our symptoms). Miryam Williamson tells me that when the fog rolls in, she feels as if there were "a veil" between herself and the rest of the world. She can distinguish between the normal forgetfulness that comes with age and what she calls "a complete, total fog." The latter can range from mildly disorienting to completely debilitating.

Cognitive problems negatively impact our family life, our work life, and our sense of self-esteem. We forget promises we make to our children, have trouble completing tasks, and wonder how we could have become so stupid. For me, writing this book is like coming out of the closet on this issue. Most of my clients never see me struggle with thoughts and words because I work exceptionally hard to put my best foot forward for them. By evening, I am exhausted by the effort. "Mom's brain doesn't work after 5 P.M.," is the way my son describes this. Because cognitive difficulties affect so many areas of our lives, we'll come back to this topic again in later chapters.

STRESS AND CHRONIC DISEASE

Often our health problems are not linked to depression but to that ubiquitous, catchall feeling, stress. More than half of the individuals in six of the seven diagnostic categories author Linda Hanner surveyed (rheumatoid arthritis, fibromyalgia, interstitial cystitis, lupus, Lyme disease, and myasthenia gravis) had been told at some point that their symptoms were not "real" or were caused by stress. Even people eventually diagnosed with multiple sclerosis received this response approximately 45 percent of the time.[19]

Many of us have been told by well-meaning friends, family members, and even doctors that we need to "de-stress" our lives. I can't tell you the number of times I have berated myself for not being able to relax or have yelled at people who suggested that I just need to take it easy. Yet, many chronic illnesses do indeed develop or worsen during a stressful time in our lives.

Emotional Stressors

Dr. James Gordon writes, "Most of the people with chronic illness whom I had treated had begun to develop symptoms after a period of prolonged and intense stress."[20]

Many of the men and women I interviewed became sick while working at stressful jobs, caring for sick parents, or juggling too many responsibilities at once. Even good stress can cause problems; I was exhausted for six months after I got married. Bob, age thirty-four and a reporter for a daily newspaper, has Crohn's disease, an inflammatory bowel disorder. "When I became seriously ill, I was incredibly stressed," Bob recalls. "I found if I could lie in bed and relax, my stomach pain felt better." He also feels much better when he is on vacation, a phenomenon that may point to the role of stress in disease.

"Symptoms that disappear on vacations are likely to arise from stressful circumstances in a person's workday life," says Dr. Andrew Weil, director of the Program in Integrative Medicine at the University of Arizona in Tucson. Further, he writes, "A healing response may immediately follow the resolution of some intolerable situation, such as ending a bad marriage or quitting a miserable job or making peace with an estranged family member."[21]

A number of the women I interviewed alluded to childhood abuse as a possible triggering event. "My theory is that while the abuse doesn't necessarily cause the disease, the internal tension it creates is a feeding mechanism for fibromyalgia," Pam believes.

Lenore, age forty-four, is certain that incest helped trigger her chronic bladder problems. When she is under stress, she clenches her pelvic muscles. "My body responds in the same way I did as a child," Lenore says. "This is a habitual response that's very difficult to break because it's all unconscious. That's different than saying it's not based on reality," she adds. "It's a very real physical reaction."

In the same way, Miryam Williamson told me, "I think a lot of us have certain habits of thought and behavior that may work against us." Because she felt insecure as a child, she developed a habit of hunching her shoulders in a defensive posture. Since learning to hold her shoulders correctly she has resolved a good deal of the pain in her upper body, which is a common site of fibromyalgia discomfort.

Though I have had certain fibromyalgialike symptoms since I was a child, I have always believed that the stress of living for many years with undiagnosed Sjogren's syndrome and being a single working mother precipitated the pain and fatigue of fibromyalgia. More recently, while writing this book, running my own business, and being a wife, mother, daughter, sister, and friend, I have frequently felt more tired and out of sorts than even I am used to being.

Physical Stressors

Sometimes a traumatic incident such as a car accident or major surgery signals the beginning of health problems or a flare-up of an underlying and perhaps undiagnosed disease. The year before she was diagnosed with lupus, Jeri fractured an ankle, broke a rib, and was in a car accident—all separate incidents. She says, "I always wondered if those events helped trigger my disease."

Recent research indicates that the sudden trauma of an automobile accident, or the cumulative damage of a repetitive strain injury, may cause posttraumatic fibromyalgia localized to the injury site.[22] In one study, nearly one quarter of fibromyalgia patients reported a precipitating injury, most often to the neck or lower back.[23]

Immune System Stressors

A number of the women I interviewed told me their physical symptoms were attributed to the stress of childbirth or having young children. Indeed, there may be a physiological basis for this idea. Because many autoimmune diseases are more prevalent in women, there is increasing interest in the role that female hormones play in the development and course of such illnesses. Recent research also suggests that fetal cells that surge into a mother's bloodstream during labor and delivery may remain long after the baby's birth and eventually trigger autoimmune diseases in women who are susceptible. Dr. Diana Bianchi, head of pediatric genetics at the Tufts New England Medical Center in Boston, believes that these cells may, at some point, be recognized as foreign, activating an attack against the woman's own tissues.[24]

When her daughter was born, Kathy Hammitt remembers being too weak to lift her into the bassinet. "The nurses would say, 'Oh, everyone's exhausted after having a baby; you have to get up and move.' But I didn't really move for a long time," Kathy says. She stopped nursing her daughter when the baby was a year and a half, and the resulting hormonal shift prompted symptoms that led to her diagnosis of Sjogren's syndrome.

For years, I berated myself for being a lazy mom; I didn't even get out of my bathrobe for six weeks after my son was born. I marveled at women who had a child one day and went to the grocery store the next. Now that I know that my pregnancy may have aggravated as-yet undiagnosed health problems, I'm not so quick to criticize my early parenting skills.

If certain chronic diseases are triggered by emotional, physical, or immune system stressors, what does this say about our role in causing and treating our illnesses? The concept of stress and its relation to physical disease is both fascinating and complex, and worthy of an extended discussion. What I learned as I pursued this topic is that although many of us with chronic disease may be adversely affected by stress, we did not consciously make ourselves sick. We can, however, use what is known about the relationship between our physical and emotional health to begin to make ourselves well.

A Closer Look at Stress

I'm certain we all have our own ideas about the meaning of the word *stress*. We might think about what causes us to feel stressed—looming deadlines, traffic tie-ups, or too many tasks and too little time. Certainly, being ill and not knowing why is stressful.

And we know how stress feels in our body—we get sweaty palms, a racing pulse, and butterflies in our stomach. We probably first discovered why this happens when we studied what is called the *fight-or-flight* response in high school biology.

The Fight-or-Flight Response.   The fight-or-flight response prepares animals to protect themselves against a perceived threat. It was named by Harvard physiologist Walter B. Cannon, who studied the effect of emotions on the autonomic nervous system. His classic work *The Wisdom of the Body* was first published in 1926.[25]

Dr. Cannon noted that during the fight-or-flight response, animals' heart rate, respiratory rate, and muscle tension increases, their intestinal activity decreases, and the pupils of their eyes dilate (increase in size). These are manifestations of activity on the part of the sympathetic nervous system, one of two branches of the autonomic nervous system that controls involuntary behavior. We saw in chapter 1 that individuals with certain chronic diseases may suffer from exhaustion of the autonomic nervous system, the result of being in a perpetual state of fight or flight.

During the fight-or-flight response, when blood pressure, heart rate, and muscle tension go up, the digestive and immune systems are depressed. "The body's healing system is put on hold," social worker Cindy Perlin explains. "That's not a big problem if you're outrunning a mugger and the stressful situation is over in ten minutes. But if you stay in that fearful mind-set all the time, specific changes in the body can lead to illness."

A Definition of Stress.   Thirty years after Dr. Cannon examined the effect of emotions on the autonomic nervous system, Canadian endocrinologist Hans Selye wrote *The Stress of Life*, which focuses on the response of the body's endocrine and immune systems to internal or external stressors.[26] Many researchers and physicians consider this to be the definitive treatise on the concept of stress.

Dr. Selye defined stress as "the nonspecific response of the body to any demand."[27] He further differentiated between *stress*, the resulting condition, and *stressor*, the causative agent. Interestingly, Dr. Selye encountered a great deal of resistance to his use of the word *stress* to connote a biological process because, he said, "In everyday English, it generally implied nervous strain."[28] Dr. Selye said that stress is more than nervous tension, is not necessarily bad, and can be avoided only by dying.

When he exposed laboratory animals to a variety of toxic substances, extreme heat and cold, and loud noises and electrical shocks, Dr. Selye discovered that their adrenal glands were stimulated, their lymphatic organs shrank, and they developed ulcers with resulting weight loss. The adrenal glands are small, triangular-shaped endocrine (hormone-producing) glands that sit atop the kidneys. They secrete hormones directly into the bloodstream to regulate metabolism and to control the body's reaction to physical and emotional stressors. The lymphatic structures, including the thymus, spleen, and lymph glands, help protect the body against infection. Dr. Selye named this initial physiologic reaction to a stressor the *alarm reaction*.

Prolonged exposure to a stressor that is not serious enough to kill an organism elicits a second phase he termed the *stage of resistance*, in which the body attempts to restore equilibrium. These first two stages of alarm and resistance represent a creative response, mobilizing the body to deal with stress.[29]

However, these benefits were lost upon continued exposure to the causative agent, Dr. Selye observed. He called this third phase the *stage of exhaustion* and remarked that its symptoms were, "in many respects, strikingly similar to those of the initial alarm reaction."[30] Dr. Selye named this entire sequence of events the *general adaptation syndrome* and speculated that a maladaptive response to stress produces what he called *diseases of adaptation*, or stress diseases, which include allergies, digestive diseases, cancer, high blood pressure, and rheumatoid arthritis.[31]

Biochemical Changes.   Dr. Selye and others have explained the biochemical reactions that take place in the human body in response to internal or external stressors.[32] During the initial alarm reaction, the body sends chemical messengers from the site of the stressed tissues to coordinating centers in the nervous system. When these messages reach the hypothalamus, that part of the brain that mediates the fight-or-flight response, the hypothalamus in turn signals the nearby pituitary or master endocrine gland. The pituitary sends messages to the adrenal cortex, the outer portion of the adrenal gland, to secrete hormones that trigger the body's stress response. This results in arousal, decreased pain, and activation of the sympathetic nervous system.

In people with fibromyalgia and related diseases, there is decreased activity of the stress system, which may contribute to fatigue, diffuse pain, and a decreased sympathetic response. This agrees with Dr. Selye, who speculated that certain diseases were due to an excess of hormones that stimulate the body's defense mechanisms, while others resulted from an excess of hormones designed to suppress this response.[33] Whether the blunted stress response shown by people with fibromyalgia and related disorders results from an underactive stress response or one that has become exhausted by overactivity, the result is the same.

"One of the things that has been shown over and over again in people with fibromyalgia and chronic fatigue syndrome is that biologically, they have an inability to respond appropriately to stressors," Dr. Daniel Clauw told me. For example, when individuals with fibromyalgia exercise, inadequate production of cortisol (hydrocortisone) by the adrenal gland, which helps suppress inflammation, has been demonstrated in response.[34] This is a particularly sore point with me. In discussions about the benefits of exercise, I always feel like the odd woman out. "Normal" people say they feel energized after exercise, and I, inevitably, want to take a nap. I asked Dr. Clauw to explain this further.

"When someone with fibromyalgia or chronic fatigue syndrome exercises, they don't produce as many catecholamines like epinephrine (adrenaline) or norepinephrine as someone who doesn't have one of these illnesses," he said. Catecholamines are a group of chemical messengers that help control the body's autonomic nervous system. "Catecholamines may allow you to exercise and not hurt or be fatigued afterwards. The reason a person with fibromyalgia or chronic fatigue syndrome hurts after exercise is not because he or she is emotionally weak."

This phenomenon is called *postexertional malaise* and is one of eight Centers for Disease Control criteria for diagnosing chronic fatigue syndrome. Of course, this doesn't mean we shouldn't exercise, but it does help explain why a twenty-minute walk might feel like a twenty-mile run. The appropriate role of exercise in treating chronic illness is discussed further in chapter 5.

Biological Programming.   Obviously, the expression "You're going to worry yourself sick" has some validity. Certainly our emotions can impact our health negatively, by triggering stress that our bodies may not be able to handle. But not everyone who experiences stress develops a chronic disease. "Most people exposed to motor vehicle accidents, emotional trauma, or viral infections don't develop a chronic illness," Dr. Clauw told me. "In that small percent that do, this response is likely biologically pre-programmed. It's something over which the individual has no control."

Clearly, we don't choose to react this way to stress. And many of the stressors we experience are not even of our own making. Those of us with fibromyalgia, for example, often react negatively to loud noises, bright lights, and uncomfortable clothing (something we call the Princess and the Pea syndrome). Becoming physically ill from such seemingly innocuous trappings of modern life as a large shopping mall or a busy airport is the result of yet another sort of stress. Sometimes I can't even identify a particular stressor, yet my heart races, my breath comes in shallow spurts, and I have trouble concentrating. It feels as if my body is running a self-test of my emergency stress response. Still, I'm relieved to know that I am not to blame for the way my body reacts.

EXAMINING BLAME

There is a fine line between accepting responsibility for our illness and taking the blame. Even if some of our attitudes and behaviors have contributed to our physical symptoms, that doesn't mean we've caused our disease.

Self-Blame

After she was diagnosed with Sjogren's syndrome, Kathy Hammitt did quite a bit of reading about the mind–body connection, and she offers this caution, "I think we have to be very careful and not go overboard with these ideas, because we can come to feel that somehow we caused our illnesses. I believe that stress contributes to disease and can make it worse, but I think it's dangerous when we start blaming ourselves for our illnesses."

Taking responsibility for getting better, rather than blaming ourselves for being sick, is key to healing, according to Dr. James Gordon. "Let's say that the way we think does contribute to our illness," he told me. "So what? That does not mean you have to blame yourself. Instead, I think this insight offers you the opportunity to do something about your health." Dr. Gordon believes that blaming ourselves for being sick is more of a problem than anything we did to contribute to our illness.

Even if we come to realize intellectually that we didn't cause our illness, we still must deal with the negative feelings that these thoughts engender. We may feel morally weak, personally defective, or ashamed. We'll examine some of these feelings further in chapter 6.

Societal Stigma

If we're not busy blaming ourselves, society may point a finger at us. Individuals afraid of confronting their own mortality may need to distance themselves from people who are ill or injured, according to Patricia Fennell. This "just world" notion (the it-wouldn't-happen-to-me concept) leads society to blame the victim of a tragedy. In turn, Fennell says, "Patients internalize the message that they caused this problem by some personal action, and therefore 'deserve' to be ill."[35]

Some of us are better than others at fending off the notion that we are to blame for being sick. I asked Miryam Williamson if she believed that some negative event or emotion in her childhood might have caused her to develop fibromyalgia. "I'm perfectly willing to believe that some of my life experiences have contributed to my pain," she told me. "But that doesn't mean that my pain is not real, or that I can just pull up my socks and make it stop."

The more we understand about the cause of our disease, the less likely we are to be hard on ourselves. We should use this knowledge to help us heal, not to become a victim, Dr. Clauw cautions. "The victim mentality is a tremendous negative factor for many chronic illnesses," he says. "When people focus on what they think caused their symptoms, whether it be an automobile accident or going to the Gulf War, they forget they are responsible for getting better."

BEGINNING TO HEAL

Responsibility is so much nicer than blame. Understanding that the connection between stress and chronic disease is more complex than the slogan "Don't worry, be happy" helps us to stop being defensive when people tell us we just need to relax. We also now have a way to begin to heal.

"If negative emotions produce negative chemical changes in the body, wouldn't the positive emotions produce positive chemical changes?" the late Norman Cousins asked rhetorically in *Anatomy of an Illness*.[36] In this well-known treatise, Cousins described his use of laughter and large doses of vitamin C to cure himself of ankylosing spondylitis, an inflammatory disease of the spine. "It makes little sense to suppose that emotions exact only penalties and confer no benefits," Cousins said. "The positive emotions are life-giving experiences."[37]

Daniel doesn't think that viewing episodes of the old George Burns and Gracie Allen show is going to cure his multiple sclerosis but he says, "Given that there are factors I cannot change, I might as well keep a positive attitude." Angela agrees. Having lived with multiple sclerosis for sixteen of her forty-nine years, she told me, "We all struggle with attitudinal change, and that *is* all in our heads." But, like me, Angela is no Pollyanna. She says, "I can't tell you I don't have days where I'm real unhappy with myself and my life. But if I dwell on these moments, I have more of them." On bad days, she makes a pot of tea and curls up with her cat. In chapters 5 and 6, we'll explore the use of humor and other types of behavioral techniques to combat the pain, depression, and isolation that accompany chronic disease. We'll also look at the need to accept and work through the negative emotions that wash over us in waves.

When thinking about the role we play in triggering or treating our specific disorders, it helps me to keep in mind the distinction some doctors make between "disease" and "illness." Alhough the terms are used interchangeably in this book, some physicians suggest that disease refers to the physical disorder we have, while illness connotes our response to the disease.[38] They believe that even when our disease cannot be cured, our illness can be healed. We take an important step toward healing when we understand the delicate balance that exists between our emotional and physical health.

3

FINDING A HEALTH
CARE PARTNER

Women want a wizard, a magical healer, a wise woman, a guru, a
friend, and a confidant all rolled into one doctor. . . . We will settle
for a competent, caring doctor who listens.[1]
MARION CROOK

The year I lost my beloved doctor was traumatic. In the first six months of
that year, I started a business, married, and moved myself and my son to
my husband's home. My sleep was erratic, my pain more intense, and my
cognitive skills marginal. But these were all surmountable difficulties. As I
settled into my new routine, my health began to improve, in part because
I could confide my troubles to my doctor. When he transferred out of state
later that year, I was devastated. The relationship I had with my doctor
was as important as any treatment I had tried.

In this chapter, we'll examine the importance of the doctor–patient relationship. In particular, we'll look at how technology and managed care
have begun to change the nature of that relationship. We'll explore what
we want from our doctors, and how we can be more effective patients. Finally, we'll take a more detailed look at the impact of managed care on the
financing and delivery of health care services. Finding a capable and caring health care partner is critical for those of us who live with chronic disease. We must remember that it is both our right, and our responsibility, to
do so.

49

EXAMINING THE DOCTOR–PATIENT RELATIONSHIP

Our attitude toward doctors may be as ambivalent as our attitude toward politicians. Some 69 percent of respondents to a 1991 American Medical Association survey claimed to be losing faith in doctors.[2] Yet other polls show that most of us are happy with our own physicians.[3] But even when we like our doctor, we may not be pleased about overall changes in patient care. In particular, though the treatment of many chronic diseases hasn't changed much in recent years, the doctor–patient relationship has undergone a profound shift.

The Doctor as Friend

From the mid-1700s to the early 1800s, physicians were not only ineffective but sometimes dangerous, Linda Hanner writes in *Healing Wounded Doctor–Patient Relationships*.[4] With such primitive treatments as bloodletting and prescriptions made from all manner of questionable ingredients, the most therapeutic intervention doctors had to offer their patients was their caring and concern. Hanner notes, "Doctors weren't so reluctant to become friends with their patients, and the caring relationship was therapeutic in itself."[5]

Doctors' roles, and their patients' expectations, began to change when better nutrition and public health practices, and later the discovery of antibiotics, led to improved treatments for common ailments. Suddenly, medicine was a respected science, and we looked to our physicians to provide a cure for every disease. In the early part of the twentieth century, for example, Paul Ehrlich helped develop antitoxins to neutralize the bacteria that caused such deadly childhood diseases as diphtheria and tetanus. "He coined the term *magic bullet* for the cures he was seeking," says Dr. James S. Gordon.[6] However, though the magic bullet approach works well for an easily identifiable and self-limiting condition like strep throat, it may be inappropriate or ineffective for many of the chronic diseases we have.

Further, Dr. Gordon notes, "This focus on the pathological processes in our patients, and on the search for accurate diagnoses, identifiable causes, and precise remedies for their diseases often tended to overwhelm our concern for them as people."[7] My doctor didn't have a cure for Sjogren's syndrome, fibromyalgia, or interstitial cystitis, but his obvious interest in my well-being allowed me to accept this fact and to replace false hope with a realistic vision of better health.

The Doctor as Technician

Many great medical discoveries have been made with the benefit of increasingly sophisticated technological tools. Reliance on technology also plays a significant role in the changing doctor–patient relationship. Physicians who used to listen to and observe a patient can order a battery of diagnostic tests. But many of us with chronic illnesses have perfectly normal laboratory results, and we may be dismissed on this basis before the cause of our problems is discovered. Conversely, a positive finding on a particular test may not be evidence of disease.

For example, Dr. Don L. Goldenberg, chief of rheumatology and director of the Arthritis/Fibromyalgia Center at Newton-Wellesley Hospital in Newton, Massachusetts, notes that magnetic resonance imaging, or MRI, detects a joint or disc abnormality in half of all people past middle age. Typically, this is from simple wear and tear, and most of these individuals have no back pain at all.[8] Unlike a CAT scan, an MRI uses powerful magnetic fields and radio waves, rather than X rays or other radiation, to provide high-quality, cross-sectional images of organs and structures within the body.

Though laboratory results can help confirm a physician's observations, the patient interview alone may be enough to make a diagnosis or to rule out certain possibilities. Eminent physician Sir William Osler, author of the classic 1892 work *The Principles and Practices of Medicine,* said that 90 percent of the time, the patient will *tell* you what the problem is.[9] As we'll see in this chapter, patients believe that one of the most important characteristics of a good doctor is the ability to listen and ask the right questions. In trying to determine whether I might have fibromyalgia, my doctor asked me if I felt rested in the morning. "Never," I told him. However, if he had asked me if I slept well, I would have said that I did. Except for occasional trips to the bathroom, I was in bed all night so I had no idea I was experiencing the nonrestorative sleep that is characteristic of fibromyalgia. He could have recommended a complex and expensive sleep study, but his careful questioning verified his suspicions.

The Doctor as Businessman

Another factor that may negatively affect the doctor–patient relationship is managed care, which we'll explore in more detail at the end of this chapter. Our doctor may become a "gatekeeper," restricting our access to specialty care, and his or her actions may be reviewed by an individual who has no medical training and whose job it is to help our health plan contain costs.

Joan O'Brien-Singer calls health maintenance organizations (HMOs), a type of managed care agency, "horrible medical options." Though two physicians supported her need for ongoing antibiotic treatment for Lyme disease, her HMO refused the request. Ironically, even had the company approved the treatment, Joan's prescription coverage would only reimburse one third of the cost of the medication she would need. There is considerable controversy in medical and scientific circles about the efficacy of long-term antibiotic treatment for Lyme disease. Although insurers may side with physicians who think that one month of antibiotics is sufficient, patients are making themselves heard. Six Lyme disease patients in upstate New York brought suit in 1997 against a major health insurance company to force it to pay for the long-term therapy they feel they need.[10] Not everyone's experience with HMOs is negative, as we'll see later in this chapter, but there is no doubt that managed care often alters the nature of the doctor–patient relationship.

The Patient as Consumer

Technological advances and managed care make it incumbent on patients to be savvy consumers of health care services. I fondly remember the days when my pediatrician made house calls and I revered him in an almost godlike way. But putting our doctors on pedestals means they are certain to fall. On the other hand, questioning their every move will leave us mistrustful and confused. What can we realistically expect of our physicians? Ideally, we want a doctor who will take the time to listen to us, work collaboratively with us, and respect the knowledge we have about our own bodies and how we want to treat them.

WHAT PATIENTS WANT FROM THEIR DOCTORS

My doctor was a lifeline for me. He was my primary care physician, my rheumatologist, and my friend. He uttered those magical words, *I believe you don't feel well.* He diagnosed me with both fibromyalgia and Sjogren's syndrome and he monitored my care, particularly the odd reactions I have to medication. My doctor read information I brought him, and we laughed together at some of the more frustrating, but funny, aspects of my health problems. I complained of transposing letters and numbers in my writing (a sign of cognitive difficulties), and he said he was glad I didn't work for a bank. When he told me that if I could keep moving all night long, my joints wouldn't be so stiff in the morning, I smiled at the implications. He wasn't perfect, and he didn't make me well, but he helped me feel better by empowering me to take care of myself. This is the kind of doctor we all want and sometimes are lucky enough to find.

In researching this chapter, I compiled a long list of what we want from our doctors, derived in part from what we don't like. The list includes such tangible assistance as education and ongoing support, and such intangible qualities as compassion, respect, and belief in our ability to get well. But all of these take time, and that seems to be in short supply.

Time

I've spent countless hours in doctors' offices over the last twenty years, and I hate to wait. Ironically, "patients" often are required to be inordinately "patient," a trait that is not my best. I have learned to bring a book or some work to read when I set off for the doctor's. But even more difficult than waiting is knowing that my visit with the doctor, when it finally comes, may be brief. Time often is in short supply in a business increasingly focused on the bottom line.

"To some extent doctors are very limited in their time commitments to the patient because of the way they get paid, and this is unfortunate," says Dr. Jill P. Buyon, associate professor of medicine at New York University School of Medicine. "Some of these managed care companies actually penalize doctors who spend more than fifteen minutes with a patient or do more than the company thinks they should." I know that I am not my doctor's only patient, but when I am in his office I want to feel as if I am.

The Ability to Listen

After many months and even years of dealing with chronic and often undiagnosed health problems, we are more than ready to tell our doctors what is bothering us. But many of us feel that our doctors can't, or won't, hear what we have to say.

Wendy Hay's legs were numb for six months after the birth of her second child. "The neurologist I saw wanted to focus on my headaches, and that's not why I was there," Wendy told me. She got angry at the doctor and decided she would deal with the numbness on her own, largely by trying to ignore it. When she nearly lost the sight in her left eye, she went to see her son's eye doctor. He took a detailed medical history and referred her to a neurologist at Michigan State University, where she subsequently was diagnosed with multiple sclerosis.

Part of the problem, according to Dr. Frederick R. Levine, a dentist in private practice in Schenectady, New York, is that doctors are taught to have an answer. He finds that he has a habit of interrupting patients as soon as the answer seems obvious. In fact, separate studies have concluded that, on average, doctors interrupt a patient after eighteen seconds.[11] "I've learned to count to three before I say something while a patient is speaking," Dr. Levine says. "There have been a few times when I hear more of what the patient has to say that I realize I didn't have the answer after all."

Willingness to Answer Our Questions

We need to be able to tell our stories to our doctor and to ask questions. But sometimes patients are afraid to question their doctors. "If a patient can't ask questions, there has got to be another doctor for that patient," Dr. Jill Buyon says. The key to managing a chronic disease, she believes, is for the patient to be able to ask as many questions as necessary, whether or not they seem stupid. She adds, "Patients should not leave the doctor's office without some understanding of why they feel the way they do and what they can do about it."

Many of us put our questions in the form of a list. Indeed, in a taped message for subscribers who are on hold, my HMO recommends that patients make the most of their visit to the doctor by preparing a list of their concerns. I take lists because I'm afraid I will forget something, especially when the visits are several months apart. Dulce is even better prepared. Having lived with fibromyalgia most of her life, though she was only recently diagnosed, she takes a folder with her questions, copies of articles and other new information she wants to discuss with her doctor, and a computer printout of her medical history, including the names and dosages of her medications.

But doctors have been trained to view written lists as a sign of psychological problems. In fact, according to Dr. Elizabeth Lee Vliet, founder and director of HER Place, women's health centers in Fort Worth, Texas, and Tucson, Arizona, "The French name for psychoneurosis is *la maladie du petit papier* (the illness of the little paper), referring to the lists of symptoms brought in by the typically *female* patients."[12] At the same time, men who bring lists, Dr. Vliet says, are seen as helpful and organized rather than neurotic or anxious.

On a more practical level, doctors may worry that a long list of questions will upset their schedule. Even physicians like Dr. Buyon, who encourages patients to bring lists, which she pastes into their charts, recommends that patients focus the questions and begin with their most important concerns first. She believes the patient should be able to accept a succinct answer and realize that the rest of the list may have to wait for another appointment.

I've started limiting my lists to three questions, which helps me focus on the most significant problems I'm having. Some doctors cringe when I pull out a list, but most are receptive to answering a limited number of questions. The doctors I really like are the ones who ask me at the end of the visit if I have any further concerns. However, this may come at a price: my urologist is particularly good at making sure his patients understand everything he has told them but he also is the physician I often wait for the longest. Still, I'm less resentful of the time I spend in his waiting room because I know I will have his full attention in the office.

Clear, Compassionate Communication

The words a doctor chooses can have great impact, both positive and negative. "A patient can walk out of a doctor's office feeling devastated or uplifted based simply on the doctor's manner or choice of words," author Linda Hanner says.[13] We feel dismissed and devalued when a doctor makes insensitive or offhand comments. When Ken Henderson told his doctor that a specialist had diagnosed him with fibromyalgia, the doctor replied, "Well, if it is fibromyalgia, there's nothing you can do about it. You just have to grit your teeth and get on about your business." Ken supports his family, despite pain in his upper body that keeps him up most nights. He hasn't had a full night's sleep in his own bed in three years. "I've thought about my doctor's comments many a night when I'm walking the floor," Ken says.

Even though we all have to learn to live with our illnesses, we don't want to be dismissed so lightly. I remember telling a gynecologist that I was having uncomfortable menstrual cramps. He assured me I didn't need to worry because the cramps were a sign that I had ovulated. I told him I wasn't worried, I just wanted something for the pain.

In addition to choosing their words carefully, we want our doctors to say what they mean. Linda Webb was sent home with an anti-inflammatory suppository for ulcerative proctitis. Her doctors told her that a month of the medication should clear it up. "By 'clear it up,' what they meant but didn't say at the time was put it into remission," Linda says. Eventually, a doctor explained to Linda that ulcerative proctitis may go into remission but that she will always have the disease. She estimates that her doctors gave her about 20 percent of the information she felt she needed on inflammatory bowel disorders. She gleaned the rest from her own research and from information provided by the Crohn's and Colitis Foundation of America, whose address can be found in the resources section at the end of the book.

We also want our doctors to tell us what they are going to do, and why. Lois Arias thought she was having a routine urological examination and was terrified that something was horribly wrong because she was in such pain after the doctor left her. She later discovered that, without telling her, the doctor had stretched her urethra, which is believed to be a possible treatment for chronic urinary tract infections. Her regular urologist was sympathetic to his colleague's method of operation. "Some doctors are afraid that if they tell the patient what they are going to do, she will be tense and clench up," he told Lois. She told her doctor, "The patient has the right to be tense."

Sometimes doctors err too far in the other direction, telling patients the worst possible implications. "Too many doctors are deeply pessimistic about the possibility of people getting better, and they communicate their pessimism to patients and families," says Dr. Andrew Weil, director of the Program in Integrative Medicine at the University of Arizona in Tucson.[14] A patient who is pessimistic about his or her recovery will have a more difficult time getting well.

Mireille was at her lowest point when a doctor offered little hope for treating her fibromyalgia. She had had a bad reaction to one medication, and he said there was nothing else he could offer her. "I thought this just couldn't be, yet here was a professional telling me it was," Mireille says. She got worse physically, and she also became quite depressed. By the time she got to another doctor, she burst out in tears in his office, something she had never done.

Miscommunication may result when we hear what the doctor says but don't understand what he or she really means. In a somewhat tongue-in-cheek look at doctor–patient communication, Dr. Timothy B. McCall, internist and author of *Examining Your Doctor,* translates doctorspeak. For example, he writes, the doctor's comment "There is no medical reason for your problems" might mean "It's all in your head (and I don't deal with that part of the body)." In similar fashion, when the doctor says, "Here's a prescription," it may mean, "Your appointment is over," and when he or she tells you, "Here's something for your nerves," it could mean, "You're getting on mine."[15]

Possibilities for misunderstanding abound on a more serious note. For example, when a doctor tries to reassure us by telling us that nothing is wrong, we may feel that we haven't been heard or that we are being accused of imagining our illness. Our doctors may be especially confused when we react dejectedly to news that all our lab results are normal. We don't want to be sick, but we would like to have an identifiable disease that can be treated easily. Though it would take my own doctor several years to diagnose both Sjögren's syndrome and fibromyalgia, he agreed to follow me on a regular basis in order to monitor my symptoms. His belief that I didn't feel well and his honesty about the difficulties of the diagnostic process helped me weather the uncertainties and fears that mark the early years of an undiagnosed illness.

Education about Our Disease

The word *doctor* derives from the Latin word *docere,* which means "to teach."[16] Dr. Timothy McCall believes this is the doctor's most important role. A doctor who skimps on patient education undermines the quality of care, he says, because patients who do not understand their condition are less likely to follow suggested treatment and to feel satisfied with the services they receive.[17]

By and large, those of us with chronic illnesses are hungry for information. We want all the details about our disease, and we want them upfront. I have file folders full of material on my various health problems, and I know from talking to others that this is not unique. I don't use this information to obsess about my health; on the contrary, the more I know, the better able I am to go about my daily life. Unfortunately, we may be left to do much of our own detective work.

Jeri learned she had lupus when she read the diagnosis on her insurance form. She has a theory about why she wasn't told. When several of her friends told her they knew people who had died from lupus, Jeri began to realize that people connect lupus with death. "I have no intention of dying from lupus," Jeri says confidently. But she suspects her doctor was reluctant to share his diagnosis, or to have her learn about the disease, because it might have confirmed any fears she might have. "As soon as my doctor told me we were going to rule out lupus, he said, 'I can tell you're the kind of patient who is going to stop at the library on the way home,' " Jeri recalls. She did, but what she found was fairly outdated. Though lupus may lead to fatal complications, new treatments and a better understanding of the disease mean that many patients today lead full and productive lives.

When we're told about the possible implications, we can be prepared for what may lie ahead, both bad and good. Daniel was "forbidden" by the neurologist who diagnosed him with multiple sclerosis to read anything about his disease. Because he knew Daniel had been researching demyelinating disorders, of which multiple sclerosis is one, the doctor said, "You're just going to find new symptoms, and you're going to suggest yourself into things." Daniel found another doctor who told him to read all that he could. Up to that point, he had been discouraged by advertisements for scooters in publications for multiple sclerosis patients. But when he began doing further research, Daniel says he was heartened to learn that 70 percent of people diagnosed with multiple sclerosis remain ambulatory. The more information he gathered, the fewer fears Daniel had.

Doctors may be reluctant to share information until they know their patients better. Kelly initially was discouraged about the lack of details her doctor provided about her lupus diagnosis. On her third visit with him, she told her doctor, "I'm the kind of person who needs to know absolutely everything. I've already bought ten books, but I wish you'd share with me what you know." Her doctor admitted he doesn't do that with everyone because some patients don't want to know a worst case scenario. When I asked my urologist whether he was considering interstitial cystitis as a possible cause of my chronic bladder problems, he said, "Oh, you don't want to have that." I assured him that though I would prefer not to have yet another chronic incurable disease, I would feel much better if I knew that's what I was dealing with.

Validation

When my rheumatologist said, "I believe you don't feel well," I immediately began to feel better. I finally had the reassurance I needed that whatever the cause of my physical problems, they were very real to me. We especially want doctors to acknowledge the emotional difficulties of living with chronic disease. Because all his test results were coming back normal, Ken Henderson told his doctor he was afraid he would die of a serious illness before they found out what was wrong with him. That's when he ended up in a psychiatric hospital. "After that I watched how I worded things to doctors," Ken says, "but that's how I felt that day." As for me, sometimes my doctor could tell just by looking at me that I was sad or depressed, and he always took the time to ask why. More often than not, my negative emotions were tied to a downturn in my physical health.

Collaboration

"If you find yourself in a medical dictatorship, try to switch to a democracy," Dr. Timothy McCall recommends.[18] We want our doctor to be our health care partner, guiding us and advising us but allowing us to have the ultimate say in our care.

"The type of doctor I value most is a collaborative doctor," Linda Webb says. "The doctor has training that I don't, but I know my body." Linda likes to be prepared, so she does her homework ahead of time. "Once I'm there, I've learned not to tell doctors what's wrong with me. It used to turn them off." Still, she adds, "I love it when a doctor says to me, 'What do *you* think it is?' " Linda's research led her to believe she had ulcerative proctitis, a diagnosis her doctor confirmed.

Because we are intensely interested in our disease and do much of our own research on possible causes and treatments, we want our doctor to be open to information we provide. If we are inclined to try alternative therapies, such as homeopathy, touch therapy, or the use of nutritional supplements, we want a physician who is willing to explore these possibilities with us.

Often, when I had regular checkups with my rheumatologist, I would take materials from the Sjogren's Syndrome Foundation. When he responded to one of my questions, my doctor would sometimes ask if the foundation material agreed with his answer. He clearly was not threatened by my reliance on other sources of information and knew that in some cases I might have uncovered more up-to-date information about Sjogren's syndrome than he had the time to do. He kept an open mind about alternative treatments, even cautiously suggesting that I might want to try certain herbal supplements that some of his other patients found helpful. He made it clear, however, that he thought most alternative treatments were costly and offered little benefit. We'll explore the debate surrounding the use of alternative versus conventional medicine and examine some of the therapies people try in chapters 4 and 5.

Today, many of us show our doctors material we have gleaned from the Internet. Dr. Jill Buyon says that whether or not she reads such information depends on how much time she has and whether it catches her eye. She says, "I can tell right away depending on the reference and how it is written whether it is useful or not. There's a lot of crap out there." Ultimately, we have to decide what to do with the information our doctors give us and that which we discover on our own. We'll discuss good ways to do this in chapter 4.

Respect

We want our doctors to respect us not only as a full partner in our care but also as a fellow human being. We don't want to be called "a wimpy old lady" or branded a "bored housewife," as some of the women I interviewed had been labeled.

Several observers have commented on the inherent inequality in the doctor–patient relationship reflected by the use of formal titles for doctors and first names for patients. Community health care nurse Marion Crook explains, "Doctors tell me that the public expects to be treated 'professionally,' and they think that introducing themselves by their title is 'professional' and calling a woman by her first name is 'friendly.' Women don't see it that way."[19]

The informality of being addressed by my first name doesn't bother me nearly as much as the ease with which some doctors imply that they know how I feel when they have no idea what I'm experiencing. Even worse, they may fail to acknowledge my discomfort at all, particularly during some painful and embarrassing medical tests. I think the film *The Doctor*, in which William Hurt plays a physician who realizes how degrading being a patient can be when he becomes sick himself, should be required viewing for every new physician. Dulce would go one step further. She thinks all doctors who treat patients with fibromyalgia should have the condition for at least six months before earning their degrees!

Respect, of course, is a two-way street. "While it is appropriate for patients to question decisions and at times be their own medical detectives, a good patient should also be honest with and respectful of doctors whose care they are under," author Linda Hanner notes.[20]

Acknowledgment of Limitations and Beliefs

When I posed a question my doctor couldn't answer, he didn't hesitate to say, "I don't know." If it was something he could determine, he would offer to look it up for me. Rather than feel annoyed at his lack of knowledge, I felt honored that he respected me enough to be honest. There are times, of course, when an answer of "I don't know" can be frustrating or even scary. For several years, I took an antimalarial drug believed to slow the progress of autoimmune diseases such as rheumatoid arthritis, Sjogren's syndrome, and lupus. I wanted to know why a drug used to treat malaria could help rheumatoid arthritis, but my doctor acknowledged that the exact mechanism is unclear. We'll discuss some specific medications used to treat chronic diseases in chapter 4.

More often than not, however, my doctor's honesty helped me better understand that medicine is as much an art as a science. He reminded me that the field of immunology is a relatively new one in medicine and that much research remains to be done. Most importantly, he never dismissed my question or concern just because he didn't know the answer. He freely admitted he couldn't explain the physiological process behind the intense fatigue I experienced, for example, but he assured me that most of his other patients who had autoimmune diseases felt tired also. He conjectured that a body that is, in essence, fighting itself, has a right to be fatigued.

In addition to wanting our doctors to know what they don't know, we want them to understand and acknowledge their own limitations and interests. According to Dr. Jill Buyon, "Some of the tension in the doctor–patient relationship may represent the insecurity of doctors about certain diseases because they don't like them, or they don't believe in them, or they really don't know how to deal with them." This is especially true for such illnesses as fibromyalgia and chronic fatigue syndrome, which are still hotly debated in medical and scientific circles. In addition, Dr. Buyon notes, "Not every physician can keep up on the literature on every disease. I really think patients have to try to get inside their doctors' heads because perhaps the disease they have is not the one their doctor is good at treating."

Ongoing Support

When it took five years to diagnose Eileen's interstitial cystitis, and another three years to find an effective treatment, her biggest fear was that her doctor would refuse to see her. But he stuck with her, and she with him. "He never gave up," Eileen says, "and that helped me get through the difficult times." For several years, her doctor would not acknowledge that she might have interstitial cystitis but he never doubted that she was in pain. He admitted that a diagnosis is often hit or miss, and he never lost his willingness to help Eileen get better.

Pam had the opposite experience. Because those of us with fibromyalgia have very individual symptoms and often experience odd reactions to medications, we must try different drugs until we find one (or a combination) that works for us. Pam couldn't tolerate the first medication her doctor prescribed because it left her feeling hungover, and she couldn't get to work in the morning. He prescribed a new drug with fewer side effects, but without a generic equivalent the medication was too expensive for Pam to continue taking. At that point, Pam says, "I feel my doctor lost interest in pursuing my treatment."

I can't tell you how many medications I have tried. Even my doctor became discouraged when most of the anti-inflammatory drugs he prescribed upset my stomach. But he never stopped looking. He would offer me samples of new medications that were supposed to be easier on the stomach, always hopeful that this time we would find one that worked. When we didn't, he proposed trying a different class of drugs to try to dampen the inflammatory response. Even though I was difficult to treat, he never made me feel that I was a difficult patient.

Belief in Our Ability to Get Well

What we want and need most of all is a doctor who is in our corner— someone who believes that we can get better, even if our disease cannot be cured. Though much of the work of healing from a chronic illness rests with those of us who are sick, a good doctor can empower us to get well. My own doctor, for example, made it clear that medically he could do little except ease my symptoms, but he never failed to show interest in my progress.

Interest in patients and belief in their disease are critical ingredients in successful treatment, according to Dr. Daniel J. Clauw. As a rheumatologist who treats many patients with fibromyalgia and chronic fatigue syndrome, he told me, "I firmly believe that if you gave someone the exact algorithm I use in taking care of patients with fibromyalgia and chronic fatigue syndrome, and they got the same group of patients I did but didn't really believe in fibromyalgia and chronic fatigue syndrome and didn't care about the patients with it, they would be much less effective in taking care of the illness." A doctor who believes we can get well provides a powerful incentive to do so.

HOW TO BE AN EFFECTIVE PATIENT

We can't be a passive participant in the doctor–patient relationship if we want to reap the benefits of a productive partnership. I've always considered myself to be fairly effective at getting the care I need, but the individuals I interviewed reminded me even more clearly that no one is as interested in my body as I am. Also, I have to admit, when I'm feeling particularly poorly, I slip into an almost childlike role with my physicians. I want them to put a bandage on my knee, kiss my forehead, and make the pain go away. If only it were that easy!

Educate Yourself

Dr. Timothy McCall advises us to "get smart." He says, "The better you understand your body and your medical problems, the better you'll be able to judge the quality of your doctor and know what to make of that doctor's advice."[21] Ultimately, our health care is in our own hands.

I was impressed by Angela's hard-won, practical advice. "Don't hesitate to do your own research," she advised me. "Go to the library and look things up. Get as informed as you can about your disease. It's your body, after all, and you have to take charge of it." Living with multiple sclerosis for sixteen years, she has seen her share of doctors, and she used to be intimidated by them. Today, she feels more like an equal partner in her own health care. "Doctors don't always know better," she says. A former librarian, Angela stays abreast of the latest news on treatments for multiple sclerosis.

We need to become knowledgeable about our health problems and possible treatment options so that we can make decisions *with* our doctor. Most likely, our doctors treat many patients with a number of different illnesses, so we can't necessarily depend on them to have the latest information on our disease. Especially when our illness is somewhat rare, we owe it to ourselves to have at least a passing familiarity with current research studies, new medication trials, and the latest publications. Information supplied by national patient advocacy organizations, such as those listed in the resources section at the end of the book, is a good place to start.

When my doctor first mentioned Sjogren's syndrome as a possible diagnosis, he also gave me the name of the Sjogren's Syndrome Foundation. I received an introductory packet of material, which included the name of a contact person in my area. Anxious to meet others with this disease, I called her, but I was discouraged to find that the local support group didn't meet anymore because members felt too sick to come out! Several years later, I became the local contact person for the foundation, fielding calls from people in my area who are newly diagnosed or who suspect they may have this disease. I always learn as much information as I impart. Likewise, many of the people I interviewed volunteer or offer financial support to such organizations as the Lupus Foundation of America, the National Multiple Sclerosis Society, and the Crohn's and Colitis Foundation.

In this increasingly electronic information age, the advent of the Internet, a worldwide network of computers that communicate with one other, has been a boon to those of us who have access to it. When I first connected to the Internet and began seeking information about my various medical conditions, I was taken aback by how much material is available. Some of it is complex, and much of it is contradictory; one person's miracle cure is another person's nightmare. Purveyors of information range from reputable national organizations to folks with an interest in a topic and the ability to post information on-line. I realized I needed to be careful how I used this vast, unregulated realm of information. My training as a journalist serves me well; I employ a healthy skepticism about miracle cures that seem too good to be true. But I was open enough to "meet" most of the people I interviewed for this book through various on-line health discussion groups. Several of these individuals have become my close friends, and their unflagging support kept me going the year I was writing this book. We'll discuss use of the Internet for information and support in chapters 4 and 6, respectively.

Ask Questions

One of the most important ways we can become educated is to ask questions, especially of our doctors. This can be frightening if we are uncomfortable questioning authority or if our doctor seems unreceptive to our concerns. Sometimes, Dr. Timothy McCall acknowledges, "A patient who asks too many questions is considered a nuisance."[22] We shouldn't let our fears stand in the way.

"You can't let medical professionals intimidate you," Angela says in her no-nonsense way. "Always, always, always ask questions. If you don't understand what doctors are telling you, ask again and again and again. Be ready and willing to weigh the side effects of medication against the possible benefits. You need to be clear and comfortable with what you're doing."

We especially should ask questions about medical tests, which may be expensive, uncomfortable, and ultimately, unnecessary. Dr. McCall suggests that if the results of a test won't change our prognosis or treatment, there's usually no reason to do it.[23] I suspect this is why my own doctor recommended against a lip biopsy to confirm a diagnosis of Sjogren's syndrome. However, our doctors may feel compelled to order tests to reassure us that all is well or to avoid potential malpractice suits. I certainly have acquiesced to many a test in order to put my own mind at ease. Most of them, of course, have come back normal. Today, I'm less likely to proceed with an invasive test when the doctor is fairly confident that nothing serious is wrong. "Invasive" is a key word; I am more willing to have an X ray taken than to let doctors examine my organs internally.

Be Assertive

Assertive patients get better. According to Dr. Andrew Weil, successful patients are those who "ask questions, read books and articles, go to libraries, write to authors, ask friends and neighbors for ideas, and travel to meet with practitioners who seem promising" and he acknowledges that such behavior may lead patients to be labeled "difficult, noncompliant, or simply obnoxious, but there is reason to think that difficult patients are more likely to get better while nice ones finish last."[24]

Mireille believes that the very notion of being the "patient" implies that you're passive—but you shouldn't be. "You wait for the machinery to turn and come up with a diagnosis and then a solution. The onus is not on the doctor to make you well," she says. "You have to be your own case manager." This is good advice that is so much easier to follow when we're not sick. I've found that the worse I feel physically, the more likely I am to let the doctor take charge. That's why I find it helpful to rehearse questions and comments I want to put to my doctors so that I can be more clear about my needs when I'm in their office, no matter how I feel that day. You can do this in front of a mirror or with your spouse or a friend. Sometimes just saying the words out loud gives you a greater sense of confidence that you have a right to take charge of your health care.

When I'm feeling particularly self-assured, I approach my medical problems as if the doctor and I are going to solve them together. That means we each weigh in with our opinions, though many of us have learned to let the doctor take the lead. Assertive is, however, different than aggressive. The doctor is not the enemy.

Even before she knew the full implications of fibromyalgia, Miryam Williamson was convinced that her nervous system somehow was involved. "There was no way I was going to go to a doctor and say, 'There's something wrong with my nervous system,' " she told me. "I'm smarter than that. You know the doctor will immediately write down 'hypochondriac.'" To Miryam, there is nothing worse than being called a hypochondriac.

Nor do we want the doctor to think we are trying to do his or her job. If I have enough information to suspect what a problem might be, I sometimes will present my findings in the form of a question, asking the doctor, for instance, if the cognitive problems I experience might be part and parcel of fibromyalgia or Sjogren's syndrome. Some doctors are annoyed at even this level of questioning, but that helps me know whether a doctor is right for me. I like those doctors who can engage in this kind of give and take.

Get Another Opinion

If we don't feel clear and comfortable about the medical advice we receive, we may want to consider getting another opinion. According to Dr. Timothy McCall, "If you have the feeling your doctor may be missing something, you may be right."[25]

The same physician has been treating Kelly for lupus since she was diagnosed nearly three years ago. Lately, she has begun to question not only whether all the medication she takes is necessary but whether the diagnosis itself is correct. "There is no test that says you have lupus or you don't, and if I don't," Kelly says, "this may be the wrong treatment." She'd like to get another opinion but she worries about hurting her doctor's feelings. "Maybe I should go someplace else, but I love my doctor and I don't want him to be offended," she says. According to the rules of her health plan, Kelly will have to ask her doctor for a referral. If she doesn't, she will have to pay out of her own pocket to seek further advice. Neither seems to be a viable option for her at this point.

A number of the people I interviewed said they wouldn't hesitate to see another doctor if they were at all uneasy about the care they were receiving. Doctors don't have time to be hurt, they assured me. I have started to listen more to my gut feelings because I have seen what happens when I don't. I was uncomfortable when an orthodontist recommended that my son have four teeth removed, but I okayed the procedure. When I found the doctor we now see, he told me the extractions had been unnecessary.

Of course, we don't always have to leave a doctor if we have problems. Kelly was discouraged when her doctor wouldn't share more information about lupus, but when she discussed her concerns with him he agreed to be more open. Like any potentially long-term relationship, the one we have with our physician may take time to develop. I've found myself in a sort of cautious dance with my new doctor, questioning whether she is clear about my medical problems and how I feel about them. More than anything, her willingness to let me do this makes me comfortable continuing to see her.

Trust Your Instincts

We can get as many opinions as our energy and our resources allow but in the end the final decision about our health care always is up to us. I like Mireille's analogy of "treating the state of your health as you treat the health of your finances. If you need information, there are specialists out there to advise you, but that's all they are doing, giving you advice." That's both reassuring and frightening. We need a trusted medical professional to be our guide as well as family and friends who can offer important feedback.

We also need to remember that choosing to do nothing is a valid option. "As a competent adult, you have the legal right to refuse any therapy a doctor recommends, no matter how advisable the doctor or anyone else feels it is or how irrational they feel you're being," Dr. Timothy McCall notes.[26] Kathy Hammitt was prepared to have surgery to have an enlarged thymus gland removed, but she elected to adopt a wait-and-see attitude. She did not develop cancer of the lymph system, as her doctors feared, and she was saved from unnecessary and potentially disfiguring surgery.

Find the Doctor Who Is Right for You

Not all doctors are created equal, and each of us has different qualities that matter most to us in a physician. Doctors and patients agree that it's important to find a good fit.

Daniel misses the doctor he left behind when he moved because that doctor had a knack of making every patient feel that he or she was the most important patient in the world. Sometimes the doctor's personality isn't that important to us. Lexiann Grant-Snider says that one of her physicians has "the personality of a kitchen cabinet, but he is an incredible diagnostician." Most important of all is to find a doctor who can treat our disease.

We can do this by getting referrals from doctors we know or from people who have the same illness. Sometimes, we find our doctors almost by chance. My favorite doctor was the only rheumatologist employed by my health plan when I needed to see a specialist for Sjogren's syndrome. Replacing him has been difficult, because he served not only as my rheumatologist but also as my primary care physician, coordinating the bulk of my health care. His replacement handles rheumatology patients only. Finding a new primary care physician was a bit of a challenge.

Before choosing the doctor I now see, I made appointments with several physicians within my health plan. Based on prior experiences, both good and bad, I can usually tell in the first visit whether a doctor is *wrong* for me. A doctor who isn't knowledgeable about or doesn't believe in my health problems, who won't take the time to answer my questions, or who seems overwhelmed by my multiple concerns raises a red flag in my mind. Interestingly, I've found that the doctor's gender matters little. I've had understanding male physicians, and I've had encounters with female physicians I would never see again (the one who said she didn't believe in premenstrual syndrome stands out in my mind). I find that it takes longer, however, to discern whether a new doctor is *right* for me. Initially, I was uncomfortable with my new primary care physician, because I soon sensed that she was going to challenge me more than I was used to. But ultimately, I think that will be good for me. She keeps after me to take better care of myself, while at the same time respecting the fact that certain stressors in my life are immutable.

Judge a Doctor's Competence

Whether by luck or hard work we usually find a doctor, but judging his or her competence can be more difficult. Individuals may have a hard time spotting a bad doctor because they may be fooled by a good bedside manner, according to Dr. Timothy McCall. "They figure a doctor who listens to them and who seems compassionate must be competent. As important as these qualities are, they don't make an otherwise incompetent physician good."[27] At the very least, he recommends finding out whether your physician is board-certified in his or her specialty. Doctors who receive board certification have completed a training program and passed a rigorous examination.

A doctor's education is important, of course, but it may be deceiving. Regardless of where doctors rank in their class, they all receive the same degree. This is why my father says he is never as interested in seeing a doctor's diploma as he is in examining his or her report card. "If I have a kidney problem, I want to know that my doctor passed those courses," Dad says.

Ultimately, finding the doctor who is right for us comes back to trusting our instincts. "Neither licensure, nor competence in a profession, nor even recommendations from a satisfied patient or trusted physician can guarantee that you'll feel good about or comfortable with a given practitioner," Dr. James Gordon writes. "It's here, in your choice of a true healing partner, that you really need to use your intuition as well as your intelligence."[28]

THE ROLE OF MANAGED CARE

Often, we are not displeased with our doctors so much as we are unhappy about the way our health care is organized and financed. More of us than ever before are in some type of managed care plan. The following discussion is based on several pieces on managed care that I wrote for the federal government, as well as on a section on managed care that can be found in Dr. Timothy McCall's book, *Examining Your Doctor*. All three sources are cited in the endnotes.[29]

The Growth of Managed Care

Enrollment in HMOs, the most common type of managed care organization, more than doubled from 1985 to 1995. Typically, managed care plans focus on prevention, offering, for example, low- or no-cost prenatal care and cancer screenings. Most studies comparing the quality of care in HMOs to that in traditional insurance plans have found them to be comparable for such diseases as high blood pressure, diabetes, and colon cancer. But disincentives in the system make it hard for many of us with chronic disease to get the care we need. At the very least, we may need to follow Mireille's advice to be our own case managers.

Fee-for-Service Medicine

Traditionally, health care insurers tended to pay whatever providers billed for their services, within certain customary costs or established limits. Cost-reimbursement encouraged high levels of use. "Fee-for-service doctors tend to order too many tests, especially ones where the profit margin is high, and to perform too many surgeries," says Dr. McCall. Also, because patients were free to select the care they deemed appropriate, no one coordinated the treatment they received from different doctors.

The Changing Doctor–Patient Relationship

Managed care has the potential to offer more comprehensive services at a lower price, but it comes with several costs. To begin with, managed care changes the usual doctor–patient relationship. Typically, an individual's primary care physician acts as a gatekeeper to determine whether referrals for laboratory tests or specialist care are medically necessary. His or her decision may be reviewed by a third party, sometimes referred to as a case manager or utilization review specialist. Routine procedures may need to be preapproved, and special treatments might require a second opinion.

Bob learned this the hard way. He went to see his primary care physician complaining of chronic diarrhea, and his doctor referred him to a gastroenterologist, who found blood in his stool. A series of tests confirmed that Bob has Crohn's disease, an inflammatory bowel disorder. More concerned about finding a cause for his symptoms than tending to administrative details, Bob didn't read the fine print on the voucher his primary care physician gave him that allowed him to see the gastroenterologist. By the time he realized that the referral had expired after six months, he had made two visits to the specialist—at $75 each—on the expired voucher. "I appealed, pleaded, and complained, but never got anywhere," Bob says. "Eventually, I gave up and paid the bill."

Capitation Financing

Managed care organizations rely to a greater or lesser degree on capitation financing. Capitation, literally "by the head," is a method for paying a provider a fixed price per person served for a specified time period and for a defined range of services. Because providers receive no more money for performing additional services, capitation can help control costs. The downside to this, of course, is that capitation may lead to underservice, particularly if cost-saving incentives are tied to a physician's salary. Some HMOs, Dr. McCall notes, "deduct the cost of some— or even all—tests, specialist referrals, and hospitalizations directly from the doctor's pay." As a result, he adds, these physicians may "favor younger and healthier patients since they require less time and need fewer tests."

Limited Access to Physicians

Finally, managed care organizations are also characterized by provider networks that limit access only to those physicians who have agreed to participate in a specific plan. If patients receive care outside of these networks, they usually must pay a higher fee. Many of us have spent the money to seek care outside of our health plan, traveling to major university centers or renowned clinics in search of help.

Round-the-Clock Care

Of course, not all our experiences with HMOs are negative. For more than fifteen years, I have been a member of a staff-model HMO, which means that my doctors are employed by the health plan and located in centralized offices. This arrangement ensures that I have access to medical care twenty-four hours a day, seven days a week. I have been to the doctor at 2 A.M., on Christmas Eve and New Year's Eve, and on frequent Sunday afternoons. The staff who answer the phones after-hours are well-trained in asking the questions they need to make appropriate referrals; in most cases, a physician assistant or nurse practitioner will call me back within the hour. Somehow, pain and fear seem intensified in the wee small hours of the morning, and I find it comforting to know that I can speak to an individual with medical training rather than just an answering service.

For primary care, I am restricted to doctors within my HMO, and specialists both inside and outside the plan must be recommended by my primary care physician. Still, that leaves me with a wide range of physicians from which to choose, and changing doctors within the plan is as easy as calling the member services office. I'm a bit put off by how large my HMO has grown since I first became a member; recently the agency merged with one of the country's largest nonprofit HMOs. Still, I have been with the organization long enough to know my way around. Most of all, I appreciate making a flat copayment for doctor's visits and recommended procedures rather than filing complicated forms and waiting for reimbursement. HMOs are not for everyone, but I have made them work for me.

Self-Managed Care

In essence, managed care becomes self-managed care. I have no trouble calling my HMO's member services office to complain about inadequate care or to inquire about coverage for a treatment I would like. But people who are new to the managed care environment or who are not used to questioning health care professionals may have a hard time learning to be their own advocate. We need to be willing to state our needs and expect that, within certain limits, they will be met. Even patients in traditional fee-for-service arrangements occasionally have problems that need to be resolved, and speaking up about them is the best place to start.

TAKING RESPONSIBILITY FOR GETTING WELL

Our doctors can teach us, advise us, and cheer us along, but the major responsibility for getting well rests with us. We may find this hard to accept in an age when medicine seems to promise a cure for anything that ails us. When we give up looking for the magic bullet, we've made a good start in the right direction.

Finding a doctor to guide our efforts is critical. We need to find one who will answer our questions, support our choices, and empower us to take charge of our health care. For our part, we need to educate ourselves about our disease and be willing to acknowledge that medicine is an inexact science and that our doctors are not our moms. Often, as we get our symptoms under control, we find that we see our doctors less, going only periodically for "tune-ups" or for ongoing support. When we have a chronic illness, time is on our side. Eventually, we learn enough about our illness and how it affects us to achieve a delicate balance between wanting our doctors to take care of us and learning to take care of ourselves.

4

NOW WHAT?

The Search for Treatments

At various times and in various places, prescriptions have called
for animal dung, powdered mummies, sawdust, lizard's blood,
dried vipers, sperm from frogs, crab's eyes, weed roots, sea
sponges, "unicorn horns," and lumpy substances extracted from
the intestines of cud-chewing animals.[1]
NORMAN COUSINS

Like Dorothy in *The Wizard of Oz*, we often discover that the wizard's
black bag holds nothing for us by way of a magic cure. With many chronic
illnesses, the best we can do is learn to alleviate our symptoms. Often, this
requires a good deal of experimentation to find the treatment that is right
for us. Recommended remedies may be expensive, inconvenient, or uncomfortable, and medications may have unpleasant or unacceptable side
effects. In search of alternatives to conventional treatment, we may turn to
such therapies as herbs, homeopathy, and therapeutic touch, some of
which are the subject of much debate in medical and scientific circles.

In this chapter, we'll examine the positive and negative experiences
that many of us have with medication, which may be the first line of defense that our physicians recommend. Sometimes, however, medication
may be inappropriate or insufficient to ease our symptoms, and we have
to explore alternatives to drugs. Some nonmedicinal therapies, such as exercise, are well documented, but many of the treatments we try are considered unconventional. We'll explore the debate between proponents of

conventional and alternative medicine and discuss how we decide for ourselves the treatments we're willing to try. In chapter 5, we'll highlight some of the specific remedies we choose as part of an individualized treatment plan.

THE MEDICATION MERRY-GO-ROUND

Like many, I have a love–hate relationship with medication. For the past ten years, I have wavered between wanting to find something—anything—that would take the edge off the pain and fatigue with which I live daily and being adamant that I don't want to take medications of any kind. I worry about putting chemicals into my system, but I sense that my own body chemistry may be aberrant and need adjusting. Sometimes I fear that the reason I take medication is to feel well enough to meet others' expectations of me, but other times I know that I choose to take medicine because *I* want to feel better. I am extremely sensitive to many medications, which makes the process of finding the appropriate balance between helpful and harmful effects both disruptive and frustrating. When the medication merry-go-round, as I call it, spins too fast, I sometimes want to get off.

A Frantic Searching Mode

When she was diagnosed with interstitial cystitis after five years of unnamed symptoms, Eileen entered what she calls a "frantic searching mode" for something to ease her bladder pain. She spent three years in that mode.

The least invasive treatment she tried was an oral medication used to coat the bladder wall. Because the drug, pentosan polysulfate sodium (brand name Elmiron®), was still undergoing clinical trials at the time, it was only available to patients on what is called a "compassionate use" basis. This meant that Eileen's health insurance company would not pay $840 for a year's worth of the medication, which received final approval from the U.S. Food and Drug Administration (FDA) in September 1996. The use of medication undergoing clinical trials is tightly regulated, and when Eileen developed a low white blood count she could no longer participate in the compassionate use program—even though the change in her blood count was believed to be unrelated to her use of the drug.

Eileen also endured lengthy treatments with several drugs that are instilled through a catheter directly into the bladder. One of these medications had to be administered three times a week for thirty weeks. Though her insurance company covered these treatments, Eileen, who was teaching fourth grade at the time, found visiting the doctor three days a week inconvenient and exhausting. With her doctor's approval, she learned to catheterize herself. "At least then I felt I was really in charge of my illness," she says. However, none of these drugs eased her pain.

Purely by accident Eileen discovered that the antihistamine she takes for sinus problems helped reduce her bladder pain to a manageable level. Because some researchers and patients believe that interstitial cystitis is aggravated by an overgrowth of mast cells, which produce histamine, antihistamines are one of the many suggested treatments. Along with changes in her diet, Eileen is able to keep her cystitis symptoms under control.

Symptomatic Relief

Though the treatments we choose for our illnesses are as individual as we are, most of us start our search in a fairly predictable way. Like Eileen, we begin, under our doctor's guidance, trying to relieve our most pressing symptoms. This might involve something as simple but effective as artificial tears for the dry eyes of Sjogren's syndrome. Artificial tears are specially formulated eyedrops that serve as tear substitutes for seriously dry eyes. Like many of the prescription medications we try, we may have to experiment to find the precise formulation that is right for us. Unfortunately, I've found that the best drops are fairly expensive, and though my use of them is medically indicated, the drops are considered an over-the-counter medication and are not covered by my prescription plan.

Addressing Pain and Fatigue

Because pain and fatigue are two of the most prevalent symptoms of many chronic diseases, most of us have tried any number of recommended medications to ease our joint and muscle aches and to improve our sleep. One common class of drugs used for this purpose is antidepressants, prescribed in much lower doses than would be effective to treat clinical depression.

Doctors typically begin by prescribing one of the older tricyclic compounds, most notably the inexpensive and widely used drug, amitriptyline (brand name Elavil®). The tricyclic antidepressants increase levels of serotonin, a neurotransmitter thought to induce sleep and reduce pain, and are frequently effective in treating fibromyalgia and related disorders, according to Dr. Daniel J. Clauw. Some of us who have autoimmune diseases also try low doses of antidepressant medication to control the pain and fatigue associated with our illnesses.

Although many people can tolerate amitriptyline, its side effects range from annoying to debilitating. Problems with dry mouth, morning grogginess, and weight gain sometimes overshadow the drug's beneficial effects.

When the upper body pain that keeps Ken Henderson awake most nights was attributed to fibromyalgia, his doctor prescribed a small dose of amitriptyline to help him sleep. "If I take enough of it to make me sleep, my mouth and throat get so dry that I can't talk, and I can't swallow," Ken says. Because of its sedative effect, amitriptyline typically is taken at bedtime. But many of us, like Mireille, can't shake the effects of the drug in the morning. "It was very evident to me that this medication wasn't going to work because I felt like a zombie," she says. When her doctor suggested that Mireille take the pills earlier in the evening, she recalls, "By about 6 P.M. my head would start to clear up, and it was time to take the medicine again. I didn't see much of that summer."

Though all tricyclic compounds are similar to one another, individuals who react poorly to one, such as amitriptyline, may be able to tolerate another, such as nortriptyline or imipramine. Unfortunately, I found several drugs in this class to be too sedating. Because fatigue is one of the symptoms that bothers me the most, I have an especially difficult time taking a drug that makes me tired even if I know this side effect might wane over time. Paradoxically, some people with fibromyalgia find that tricyclic medications keep them up rather than help them sleep, notes Miryam Williamson in *Fibromyalgia: A Comprehensive Approach*.[2] Indeed, one of my doctors has said that while research reveals the most common reactions that a group of individuals may experience from a medication, all bets are off when it comes to applying statistics to any one individual. Further, my doctors know that if anyone is likely to have an unusual response to a drug, it will be me!

A Newer Class of Drugs

Some of us who can't tolerate the tricyclic medications may be helped by the newer class of antidepressants called selective serotonin reuptake inhibitors, or SSRIs, which inhibit the reuptake of serotonin and allow it to exert a longer-lasting effect. These drugs may be especially helpful for individuals who have concurrent depression, according to Dr. Daniel Clauw. Prozac® (fluoxetine) is the most well-known drug in this class, but many people take its cousins Paxil® (paroxetine) and Zoloft® (sertraline). The major benefit of the SSRIs is their lack of sedation, but for some individuals these drugs may be too stimulating and exacerbate sleep disturbances, according to Drs. Robert M. Bennett and Glenn A. McCain.[3] Dr. Bennett is chairman of the Division of Arthritis and Rheumatic Diseases at Oregon Health Sciences University, where he directs the fibromyalgia treatment program, and Dr. McCain is associate director of the Pain Therapy Center in Charlotte, North Carolina. The SSRIs also may cause dry mouth and are associated with sexual dysfunction.

The Stigma of Antidepressants

For those of us who are too sleepy when we take tricyclic antidepressants and too stimulated on the SSRIs, doctors frequently prescribe small doses of both types—an SSRI to be taken in the morning and a tricyclic for bedtime. This type of therapy worked well for me physically, though I have a philosophical problem with taking one medication to counter the effects of another. Also, for years I was opposed to taking any antidepressant medication at all because of the stigma I felt was attached to it. This feeling persisted even though, as a mental health writer, I know that depression is as biological a disorder as Sjogren's syndrome.

"People often resist the notion of taking a drug classed as an antidepressant, believing that it will label them as having a psychiatric disorder rather than a physical disorder," Miryam Williamson writes.[4] I decided to give antidepressant medication a serious try when an unrelenting spell of pain and fatigue began having a negative impact on my work and on my family. This meant being willing to undergo the trial-and-error process of finding the exact combination of drugs in the right dosages taken at the optimum time of day to alleviate my symptoms with the fewest negative side effects. Because I felt so sick, I was highly motivated to do so, but that didn't make it easier to bear sleepless nights and stomach upset before I settled on the drugs that worked for me.

Unfortunately, the benefits of antidepressant therapy may wane over time, according to Drs. Bennett and McCain. One study of fibromyalgia patients concluded that after two years of treatment there was no difference in therapeutic effect between antidepressant and placebo.[5] Also, certain side effects may become worse over time. Though I was fairly comfortable on a particular combination of drugs for nearly a year, I had to stop taking one of the medicines when my urologist feared it was causing urinary retention, a less common but potential side effect of antidepressant medication. Ironically, I started a new medication, with all the uncertainties that implies, while I was revising this chapter. All my feelings about medication, both good and bad, resurfaced, reminding me that finding an appropriate treatment for chronic illness isn't like taking a course and passing the final exam, never to study the subject again. Rather, it's more like being certified in a profession that requires continuing education and relicensure on an ongoing basis.

Anti-Inflammatory Drugs

To control pain many of us try the so-called nonsteroidal anti-inflammatory drugs, or NSAIDs, including over-the-counter remedies like aspirin and ibuprofen, as well as a wide range of prescription medications in the same category. NSAIDs typically are used to dampen the inflammation that causes joint pain in such diseases as rheumatoid arthritis, Sjogren's syndrome, and lupus. However, although NSAIDs can take the edge off severe pain, they may not be helpful for the chronic pain of such illnesses as fibromyalgia, according to Drs. Bennett and McCain. Also, many of us are bothered by stomach upset. I couldn't tolerate any of the NSAIDs my doctor prescribed to control inflammatory arthritis, even with the addition of medicine to soothe my stomach. Since my arthritis is mild, I made the choice to have minor pain in my joints rather than a gnawing ache in the pit of my stomach. Frequently, those of us with chronic disease must "choose" between our symptoms and the side effects of medication designed to relieve them.

Disease-Modifying Agents

When symptomatic relief doesn't help or isn't well tolerated, our doctors may turn to a second line of defense often referred to as disease-modifying agents. These medications appear to have an effect on the underlying disease process. Two of the more common medications used to slow the progress of rheumatic diseases, including rheumatoid arthritis, Sjogren's syndrome, and lupus, are the antimalarial drug hydroxy-chloroquine (brand name Plaquenil®) and the anticancer drug methotrex-ate, both of which are believed to have a broad, anti-inflammatory effect.

Most of the people I spoke with who have rheumatic diseases have tried Plaquenil or its generic equivalent at one time or another with vary-ing results. My arthritis symptoms seemed to subside during the three years I took hydroxychloroquine, though often it is hard to pin a cause and effect on any one treatment since many illnesses will remit and flare for no apparent reason. Also, though my arthritis has never been as bad as it was before I took this medication, many patients experience a recur-rence of symptoms when a second-line agent is discontinued.[6] Individuals who take hydroxychloroquine are advised to visit an ophthalmologist reg-ularly because one of the potential side effects of this medication is loss of peripheral vision.

To reduce exacerbations of multiple sclerosis, Wendy Hay uses a syn-thetic interferon, interferon beta-1b (brand name Betaseron®). Natural in-terferons are produced by the body to fight viral infections and other stimuli. The drug is administered by subcutaneous (under the skin) injec-tion every other day. Another synthetic interferon used to treat multiple sclerosis is delivered by intramuscular injection once a week, but this re-quires a much larger needle, according to Wendy. She chose the smaller needle rather than the less frequent but deeper injections. She has learned to self-administer the drug and does not hide it from her sons, ages eight and four. Their reaction is matter-of-fact. They think, " 'Oh, there's Mom shooting up again,' and they run right by," Wendy says. "I decided I'd never hide it from them because they were going to see the needles and the medication, which I keep in the refrigerator."

Steroids

Many of us find that even second-line agents don't quell our symp-toms. If our situation is serious enough, doctors may bring out what I think of as the "big guns"—powerful drugs designed to reduce inflam-mation and, at higher doses, to suppress an overactive immune system. Typically, these are the corticosteroid drugs, which are similar to the cor-ticosteroid hormones produced by the body's adrenal gland. One of the most commonly used drugs in this class is prednisone.

Daniel found out how wonderful steroids can be the first time he was hospitalized for complications of multiple sclerosis. "That was the best vacation I ever had in my life," Daniel says. "I had no idea how jazzed up I was until I realized I had read six books, learned a new computer language, and took fifty pages of handwritten notes, all in a week. You can't use steroids very often," he acknowledges, "because they're powerful drugs."

Bob had a similar reaction to prednisone used to control his Crohn's disease. "I miss the prednisone sorely when I'm not on it," Bob says. He was taking forty-five milligrams daily of a drug that comes in as small a dosage as one milligram tablets. "It doesn't just work on your digestive system," Bob says. "All my pain vanished. I got by on five to six hours of sleep a night. I was energetic and productive. I was experiencing side effects, including mood swings and weight gain, but I didn't care because I felt so good." Eventually, Bob's doctor suggested he wean himself off the drug. Patients must taper off prednisone slowly because sudden withdrawal of corticosteroid drugs may cause serious illness or death.

As the drugs become more powerful, so too do the side effects. Prolonged use of steroids may produce significant weight gain and increased risk of diabetes, osteoporosis, high blood pressure, and cataracts. I took prednisone for three months, and I have hidden away a family picture taken during this time because I'm self-conscious about how swollen my face looked. My mother had severe osteoporosis worsened by a daily dose of prednisone to control asthma, and she had two cataracts removed.

Weighing the Risks

Taking a medication that helps with one symptom but makes another worse is not uncommon. The antidepressant medication I take exacerbates the dry mouth of Sjogren's syndrome. Antibiotics are another culprit. Because they kill good bacteria as well as bad, prolonged use of antibiotics leaves us susceptible to an overgrowth of fungi. For the nearly eighteen months that I tried various antibiotics to ease my bladder symptoms, I was rarely without a vaginal yeast infection.

Sometimes it becomes difficult to tell the side effects of a medication from the symptoms it is designed to treat. I have very little patience with medicines that make me sleepy or upset my stomach, since I'm likely to feel this way anyway. Yet when I complain to doctors about these side effects, they remind me that these problems are just as likely to be symptoms of my disease.

An Expensive Solution

Depending on the type of prescription coverage we have, buying drugs we may not tolerate can be an expensive proposition. I have learned to ask my doctors to write a small prescription for a new medication, with refills if I find I can take it. In addition, pharmacies will fill a portion of a prescription if you request this. Doctors frequently get samples of new drugs from pharmaceutical company representatives, and your physician may be willing to give you one or two packages to get you started on a new prescription.

When Linda Webb's ulcerative proctitis didn't improve after a month of anti-inflammatory suppositories, her gastroenterologist prescribed something called a retention enema. As its name implies, Linda had to hold this medication in her system for a period of time. "I kept waking up because I was afraid I wasn't going to be able to retain the medicine," Linda says. "Also, I didn't realize there was sulfa in it, and I'm allergic to sulfa." Her doctor prescribed a month's worth of medication, and Linda asked the pharmacist to fill half the prescription, at a cost of $250. She has twelve of the enemas left. Linda says, "I have so many drug sensitivities, now I go home and research the medication before I fill the prescription."

Pam found relief for her fibromyalgia symptoms but couldn't afford to take it. She missed work repeatedly when an antidepressant she was taking left her too sleepy to get up in the morning. Her doctor switched her to a less sedating but more expensive medication that kept her pain in check and didn't leave her feeling hungover. However, Pam could not afford to pay $200 a month out of pocket and wait to be reimbursed by her insurance company for 75 percent of the drug's cost. She "chose" to go without.

A Sense of Desperation

When we don't feel better despite everything we try, we may begin to feel a bit desperate. A single woman who had never had children told me she was willing to try a medication her doctor recommended even though it might render her infertile if it would relieve her myriad, undiagnosed symptoms. Unfortunately, she says, the medicine made her so sick she was unable to take it.

Lois Arias spent roughly $5,000 out of pocket over the course of a year trying to relieve the pain and discomfort of interstitial cystitis. The treatments she tried included two six-week courses of a medication instilled directly into the bladder. Still, money couldn't buy relief. Finally, Lois turned to an experimental antibiotic treatment that she says has left her 85 percent pain free.

Though it involves the use of recognized antibiotics, the treatment Lois uses is not condoned by the American Medical Association or the Interstitial Cystitis Association because the theory on which it is based is controversial. The protocol was developed by a microbiologist who believes that interstitial cystitis is caused by bacteria. Many in the medical and scientific communities dispute this notion, and they worry that long-term antibiotic use will render bacteria resistant to these drugs. Lois's doctor does not believe in this treatment and, she says, many of her fellow sufferers won't try it.

"I told my doctor I was willing to take the responsibility for this treatment," Lois says. "He doesn't have to believe in it, but I do need him to write the prescriptions." Despite his own misgivings, her doctor prescribes the recommended antibiotics because he has seen Lois improve with this treatment. Lois's husband has been treated with antibiotics as well, on the theory, also unproven, that interstitial cystitis may be sexually transmitted.

When it feels that nothing we've tried has worked, or we're unhappy with the costs or side effects of medication, we may reach beyond the boundaries of mainstream medicine for treatment and advice. After years of living with lupus, Jeri says she is willing to do whatever it takes to get well. "If standing in the yard in a pile of cow manure would make me well, I'd do it." Short of that, she has had some success treating her symptoms with homeopathy, meditation, and imagery, some of the alternative therapies we'll discuss in chapter 5.

But desperate people get into trouble, according to Dr. Jill P. Buyon. Like many scientifically inclined physicians, she worries that patients may eschew traditional therapies that are proven to help in favor of alternative remedies that may be expensive, useless, and even dangerous. The debate between proponents of conventional medicine and alternative treatments often is confusing and contentious. But, as we'll see in the next section, it is never dull.

CONVENTIONAL VERSUS ALTERNATIVE TREATMENT

I infuse myself into this debate with some trepidation. There was no topic I researched about which people felt more passionate. Many so-called flame wars, the electronic equivalent of a nasty argument, erupt on Internet discussion groups when proponents of a particular treatment, either conventional or alternative, refute their critics. I suspect the following discussion may make both sides unhappy. My attempts at some level of journalistic objectivity almost certainly will offend the *opponents* of alternative medicine who would like the media to spread the word about how dangerous these treatments can be.

When I spoke to Dr. Stephen Barrett, a retired psychiatrist and board member of the National Council Against Health Fraud, he chided me for my attempt to examine both sides of this issue. "'Nonjudgmental' attitudes of this sort, which are common among reporters, help explain why sensational health-related claims frequently appear without challenge in the media," Dr. Barrett says.[7] That I even spoke to Dr. Barrett, a self-proclaimed "quackbuster" and one of this country's most outspoken critics of alternative medicine, most definitely will cause some *adherents* of alternative care to question my motives.

Still, this is such a crucial topic for those of us with chronic disease that I'm going to plunge ahead. I know that I am not alone in wanting to weigh all sides of an issue, so that I can make an informed decision based on my knowledge, values, and beliefs. I'm confident that the following discussion will at least be reasoned, if not conclusive. Following this section, we'll look at how some of us decide for ourselves what to believe.

Some Common Ground

Despite the fervent and often opposing beliefs they hold, proponents of conventional and alternative medicine typically cede several important points to one another. For example, even those in the forefront of the movement to bring alternative therapies into the mainstream agree that conventional medicine has a critical role to play. Dr. James S. Gordon, who was trained at Harvard, writes that he would not rely on an alternative approach "if my blood pressure were so high that I might soon have a stroke, or if my system were overwhelmed by a bacterial infection, or if I were bleeding from an ulcer-ravaged large intestine. This is where Western medicine shines."[8] Norman Cousins' book *Anatomy of an Illness*, which describes how the author used large doses of laughter and vitamin C to cure himself of ankylosing spondylitis, a degenerative arthritis of the spine, is a call to arms for many who espouse alternative therapies. Still, even Cousins noted, "It would not be in the interest of the holistic health movement to regard the medical profession as the enemy."[9]

Vocal critics of alternative therapies do acknowledge that people get better on them, though they are reluctant to credit the treatment as the source of improvement. "I do not doubt that some people are helped by alternative treatments, but it is very difficult for an individual to know whether something has worked or whether they have gotten better because of the passage of time," Dr. Stephen Barrett told me.

Opponents also concede that alternative practitioners may be particularly good at giving patients what they want. Dr. Barrett and William T. Jarvis, president of the National Council Against Health Fraud, note, "The practice of healing involves both art and science. The art includes all that is done for the patient psychologically. The science involves what is done about the disease itself. . . . In a contest for patient satisfaction, art will beat science nearly every time." Practitioners of alternative medicine, the two men believe, "are masters at the art of delivering care."[10] This rings true with me. I don't understand the science of massage, but I do know that my massage therapist treats me as her most important client when I am in her office.

Finally, even the most virulent critics of alternative medicine do not believe its promoters intend to deceive. According to Dr. Barrett, "In most cases, the people who are practicing alternative medicine believe in it, so I wouldn't use the word *fraudulent* when someone has an honest but mistaken belief." These points aside, there is a great deal of disagreement in the ranks, beginning with the issue of nomenclature.

A Rose by Any Other Name

No one, it seems, is happy calling alternative medicine *alternative*. "It's a new name for snake oil," *New England Journal of Medicine* executive editor Dr. Marcia Angell told *New York Times* science writer Gina Kolata. "The very name 'alternative medicine' is Orwellian newspeak, implying that it is a viable option."[11]

Proponents of alternative medicine don't like the word *alternative* for other reasons. They note that many so-called alternative therapies are considered traditional medicine in large parts of the world, and that what we think of as traditional medicine is a relatively new phenomenon.

We should stop using the phrase "alternative medicine" altogether, according to Dr. James Gordon. "I think what we are really talking about is part of the *evolution* of medicine," he says. In his book *Manifesto for a New Medicine*, Dr. Gordon proposes a new medicine paradigm that blends ancient wisdom and modern techniques to create a less toxic, more compassionate system that teaches people how to take care of themselves. Self-awareness, relaxation, meditation, diet, and exercise should be the key ingredients in patient care, he believes, with surgery and drugs used as treatments of last resort.

To differentiate it from alternative treatment, the care we receive from our family doctor often is called conventional medicine, but that also is a misnomer, Dr. Stephen Barrett believes. "We do not use the word *conventional* because our work is not based on convention," he told me. Dr. Barrett prefers the term *scientific* medicine, meaning that its methods are reliable and reproducible from one practitioner to another.

Interestingly, the term *holistic*, sometimes used to refer to alternative medical practices or to a blend of conventional and alternative treatments, may be falling out of favor because of overuse or misuse. The term, from the Greek word *holos*, meaning "whole," was coined in 1926 by Jan Christiann Smuts, the first prime minister of South Africa, who said that the whole is more than the sum of its parts.[12] "Holistic is in the same category of adjectives as 'new,' 'improved,' and 'organic,'" writes California physician Jeff Kane, author of *Be Sick Well*. "The problem is that words and the realities they represent can be shockingly disparate. I've never met a medical doctor who didn't claim to treat 'the whole patient.'"[13]

Who Seeks Alternative Care?

If statistics can be believed, many of us are looking outside our doctors' offices for help. In a 1997 survey of trends in alternative medicine use in the United States since 1990, principal investigator Dr. David M. Eisenberg of Boston's Beth Israel Deaconess Medical Center reported that total visits to alternative medicine practitioners increased by almost 50 percent from 1990 and exceeded visits to all U.S. primary care physicians.[14]

In 1997, four in ten Americans used at least one form of unconventional medicine, according to Dr. Eisenberg. We spent $21.2 billion for services provided by alternative medicine practitioners, $12.2 billion of which we paid out of pocket. The majority of us used unconventional therapies to treat chronic problems such as back pain and headaches, and fewer than 40 percent of individuals who used alternative treatments told their doctors they had done so.

For purposes of the telephone surveys they conducted in 1991 and 1997, Dr. Eisenberg and his colleagues defined alternative medical therapies as interventions "neither taught widely in U.S. medical schools nor generally available in U.S. hospitals."[15] These included such techniques as acupuncture, chiropractic, and homeopathy. However, Dr. Stephen Barrett and his colleagues at the National Council Against Health Fraud have criticized the investigators for also including what they believe to be medically appropriate approaches, such as weight-loss programs and self-help groups, as well as some treatments that may or may not be appropriate depending on the circumstances, such as biofeedback, hypnosis, massage, and relaxation therapy. Because of these methodological problems, Dr. Barrett believes that the reported totals are meaningless.

Still, the investigators' recommendation that medical schools include information about unconventional therapies in their curriculum appears to have been heeded. As of February 1997, 38 of the country's 125 medical schools, including Harvard, Yale, and Johns Hopkins, offered courses in alternative medicine, according to the Rosenthal Center for Complementary and Alternative Medicine at Columbia University. The Rosenthal Center maintains a regularly updated list of such courses on its Web site. Details on how to access this information are included in the resources section at the end of the book.

Physicians themselves also may be interested in seeking alternative care. According to an article that appeared in *Life* magazine in September 1996, more than half of family physicians regularly prescribe alternative therapy or have tried it themselves.[16] Though most of my physicians are fairly conservative, my new primary care physician teaches and practices a self-awareness exercise that is similar to meditation, and my urologist sometimes refers clients to his wife, a physician trained in Aruveydic medicine, a traditional Indian healing system.

Further, people with health problems are not the only ones interested in pursuing alternative medicine. Many insurance companies and HMOs are jumping into the fray. HMOs in particular may be looking to save costs on less expensive alternative care and increase membership by attracting patients who demand such services. In October 1996, Oxford Health Plans, serving 1.9 million members in five Northeastern states, became the first major health insurer to offer subscribers a network of alternative providers. Without a referral from their primary care provider, Oxford members may see acupuncturists, naturopaths, massage therapists, yoga instructors, nutritionists, dieticians, and chiropractors who meet the health plan's strict credentialing requirements. The company also offers a discount mail order service for vitamins and herbal supplements.[17]

What Are We Hoping to Find?

"The reason people go to nonmedical practitioners is simple: they want to feel better," Dr. Edward W. Campion, deputy editor of the *New England Journal of Medicine*, wrote in a commentary that accompanied publication of Dr. Eisenberg's 1991 survey.[18] That's the simple truth, but it bears explaining further. When we seek alternative care, we are looking for less toxic remedies, caring providers, and the opportunity to control our own recovery.

A Different Approach to Healing.   To begin with, many feel that conventional medicine has little to offer those of us with chronic disease. Dr. James Gordon spells out in detail what he believes to be the shortcomings of biomedicine:

> It is inadequate to explain the origins or treat the consequences of the chronic illnesses, the disabilities, and the distresses that afflict more than 80 percent of those who seek medical attention. Its overuse and misuse has produced a deadly host of mutated bacterial and viral lifeforms, and an epidemic of iatrogenic—physician-and-treatment-caused—illnesses. Its economic cost—almost one trillion dollars a year and close to 15 percent of our gross national product—has become insupportable. Even its metaphors of regulation and conquest, which once seemed fitting and hopeful, now strike increasing numbers of us as both grandiose and inappropriate.[19]

Those of us who use alternative medicine don't usually start there. We've gone the conventional route first. I've been getting a regular massage for the last several years, but I sought that as an answer to ongoing muscle pain only after years of various medications proved ineffective. Interestingly, as the benefits of massage become more clear many physicians consider it a mainstream practice, though one that few insurers will cover.

Dr. Stephen Barrett believes that blaming the rise in alternative medicine on the failures of scientific medicine is like "considering the success of astrology the fault of astronomy. Some people's needs exceed what ethical, scientific health care can provide."[20] He accuses the media with starting a flood of interest in alternative medicine. But if those of us with chronic disease merely followed the latest fad, our search to find an appropriate treatment would be easy.

For my part, I'm attracted by the less invasive and more personalized nature of many alternative practices, but I'm ambivalent about entrusting my health care to a practitioner whose methods and theories I don't quite understand (not that I pretend to know much about medicine, either). Though I have no philosophical problem with alternative medicine, I tend to rely on conventional treatments for the bulk of my own health care. I suspect my attitudes were formed at an early age, when my pediatrician, who made house calls, seemed both compassionate and authoritative. But I've had to accept the fact that relying on my doctors' advice and expecting them to make me well are two very different things. My forays into alternative care, however limited, have taught me that the bulk of the responsibility for getting well always rests with me. This, I think, is the great contribution of alternative medicine to health care today and a large part of its appeal to those of us with chronic disease. After years of interventions that have been done *to* us, we welcome the opportunity to choose a treatment, like meditation or biofeedback, that allows us to do *for* ourselves.

A Different Kind of Provider.   Even more than looking for a different kind of treatment, many of us seek alternative care because we are looking for a different kind of treatment provider. We seek a "better human connection," says Dr. Timothy B. McCall, the author of *Examining Your Doctor.* Dr. McCall believes the rise in popularity of alternative practitioners, "in part reflects the fact that they provide what many conventional physicians do not, time and attention—whether or not their treatments are otherwise effective."[21] We want more than a quick visit in a sterile examining room that ends with a prescription or a polite dismissal.

To help treat her lupus symptoms, Jeri sees a physician who practices homeopathy. "He asks about my food desires, my temperament, and my symptoms, and he never doubts anything I say," Jeri says. "He writes it down as fact. I would see him just for that. He treats me as a partner in the healing process." We'll explore Jeri's experience with homeopathy in more detail in chapter 5.

Health Care Options.   Finally, those of us with chronic disease want to keep our options open. "Of all the mistakes made by physicians that hurt the American people, one of the most powerful and pervasive is their erroneous belief that they alone practice medicine," note the directors of the People's Medical Society, a consumer health organization.[22] Indeed, many traditional forms of medicine have survived for centuries, and some of their practices have become the foundation of today's scientific medicine. It would be more useful, according to nurse Marion Crook, author of *My Body*, "if doctors realized that they were part of a medical system that provided good service and good information in a narrow area of health care."[23]

Clinical social worker Cindy Perlin understands the need to offer her clients a variety of alternative therapies. She does so in the hope that "maybe they can relax rather than take high blood pressure medication the rest of their life. Maybe they can learn to warm their hands and not have to take migraine medicine. Maybe they can get off narcotics for pain or not have to take them at all."

Does Alternative Medicine Work?

What we call alternative medicine, how many of us use it, and why we do so is of little consequence if the treatments don't work. This is the point on which the critics and the true believers most vehemently disagree. Alternative medicine, Dr. Stephen Barrett says, "will take your money and break your heart."[24] Jeri doesn't see it that way. She was able to reduce the number of drugs she was taking, most of them aimed at controlling her lupus, from ten a day to two—one for a thyroid condition and one to help prevent osteoporosis.

The discussion about whether alternative medicine works seems to hinge on two major points—the validity of research being conducted and the role of the placebo effect. "Being a scientist means having an open mind and looking critically at the evidence," Dr. James Gordon told me. The evidence for the effectiveness of selected alternative treatments includes the following research findings:

- Harvard cardiologist Herbert Benson, who demonstrated that different kinds of meditation and prayer can produce what he calls a "relaxation response," subsequently found that regular relaxation can decrease levels of stress hormones, improve immune system functioning, diminish chronic pain, improve mood, and enhance fertility.[25]

- Tiffany Field and her colleagues at the University of Miami's Touch Research Institute demonstrated that premature infants given regular massages gained weight faster and were able to leave the hospital sooner than those babies who received only customary hospital care.[26]

- Dr. Dean Ornish, director of the Preventive Medicine Research Institute at the University of California School of Medicine in San Francisco, has demonstrated that coronary heart disease can be reversed by a comprehensive program that includes an extremely low-fat diet, aerobic exercise, meditation, group therapy, and smoking cessation.[27]

- Women with metastatic breast cancer (cancer that has spread to some other part of the body) who participated in therapeutic support groups designed by Dr. David Spiegel, director of the Psychosocial Treatment Laboratory at Stanford University School of Medicine, lived an average of eighteen months longer than patients who were not in the groups. Group activities included such techniques as relaxation and self-hypnosis.[28]

- Cardiologist Randolph Byrd divided patients in a coronary care unit at the University of California Medical Center into two groups, one of which was prayed for daily by a group of individuals who knew only the patients' first names and their medical condition. Patients who were prayed for had significantly fewer cardiac arrests and fewer episodes of congestive heart failure and pneumonia, and spent less time in the coronary care unit, than the patients who received medical care alone.[29]

Double-Blind Studies.   I like knowing that a treatment I am considering has shown positive results. To many scientists, however, the only evidence that is worth looking at is that derived from a controlled, double-blind study, and they point out that some investigations of alternative methods do not fit this model. In a controlled study, also called a randomized controlled trial (RCT), study participants are divided into two groups. One group gets the treatment being studied and the other receives a placebo (an inert substance) or another treatment to which the first is being compared. Neither investigators nor participants know which group receives which treatment. The codes are broken at the end of the study when the results are analyzed.

Dr. James Gordon acknowledges that RCTs have become the gold standard of clinical research, but he believes they work best for simple interventions with easily definable disease states. This approach has limited effectiveness for techniques in which the practitioner cannot be "blinded" to what he or she is doing, such as acupuncture or chiropractic, or those that depend on active patient participation, such as exercise and visual imagery.[30]

In addition, Dr. Gordon told me, some things can't be measured scientifically. "How do you measure God's grace?" he asked rhetorically. But he thinks many alternative therapies can be studied by using methodologies appropriate to the subject under investigation. Such techniques include outcome studies, in which investigators interview patients or measure their blood chemistry without interfering in any obvious way with the treatment being studied.

Not every treatment that has yet to be proven is suspect, Dr. Stephen Barrett told me. He defines as an *experimental alternative* any treatment that has "a scientifically plausible rationale or a reasonable amount of data suggesting it might be useful and is undergoing study with a clear-cut protocol." Many new treatments begin as experimental alternatives.

National Center for Alternative Medicine.   To research and evaluate alternative medical practices, Congress mandated that the National Institutes of Health (NIH) establish an Office of Alternative Medicine, now called the National Center for Complementary and Alternative Medicine (NCCAM). Since its inception in 1992, NCCAM has become a lightning rod for both sides of this issue. Many proponents look to NCCAM to make the results of research on alternative medicine more readily available. But some alternative practitioners worry that government oversight means their work will be regulated or suppressed.

By far the harshest critics of the office are those who believe that alternative medicine cannot, or should not, be studied at all. "Some academic scientists say the office follows questionable standards and is awarding grants for dubious studies," says *New York Times* science writer Gina Kolata.[31] In an op-ed piece questioning the use of tax dollars to support this venture, two scientists contend, "The real question is not whether alternative medicine is good science but whether it is science at all." They lament the fact that alternative medicine "has come to be cloaked in a mantle of NIH respectability."[32]

NCCAM has produced a voluminous report titled *Alternative Medicine: Expanding Medical Horizons*, which examines, but does not endorse, such diverse practices as Chinese medicine, bioelectromagnetics, art therapy, and therapeutic touch. Information about how to obtain a copy is included in the resources section at the end of the book. The office also established ten specialty research centers, at a total cost of $9.7 million, for three-year studies of various alternative interventions.

Testimonials.   In lieu of research data, alternative practitioners often rely on testimonials from satisfied patients to spread the word about their successes. "It is this kind of 'I went in there on a cane and I came out walking freely' personal recommendation that creates interest, respect, and acceptance by people in the community," community health care nurse Marion Crook writes. "Alternative medicine establishes its own credibility."[33]

But sometimes testimonials give alternative medicine a bad name. Many critics look askance at such evidence, fearing that testimonials may be falsified or contributed by people with a financial interest in the product. In addition, according to Dr. Stephen Barrett, "Nobody knows what percentage of the people taking a treatment achieve the same results, and nobody knows whether people actually had the disease they say they had." Unsolicited advice sometimes makes me uneasy; I value most the recommendations of people whose counsel I seek. Ever the independent soul, I like to gather all the evidence myself before making a decision.

The Placebo Effect.   Most people who use unconventional therapies get better because chronic diseases have natural periods of remission, Dr. Barrett says, refuting a popular notion that alternative treatments work by exerting a powerful placebo effect on the patient. "Nobody has demonstrated that alternative treatments produce a placebo effect that is more effective than doing nothing."

The word *placebo* is from the Latin verb meaning "I shall please." Placebos are inert substances that nineteenth-century physicians used more to please their patients than to benefit them, according to Dr. Gordon. In modern usage, placebos are used as controls in studies of new medications. Though individuals given a new drug under study are expected to show the most dramatic improvement, often people who receive a placebo get better as well. A review of medical literature indicates that, regardless of the drug being tested or the condition being treated, placebos are, on average, 35 percent as powerful as drugs that are known to be effective.[34]

Faith in a treatment or the person giving it can be strong medicine, many believe. The fact that a placebo has no physiological effect if a person knows it is a placebo, Norman Cousins wrote, "confirms something about the capacity of the human body to transform hope into tangible and essential biochemical change."[35] He noted that several doctors suggested that his treatment of ankylosing spondylitis with laughter and vitamin C had been nothing more than "a mammoth venture in self-administered placebos." But he said this theory didn't bother him at all. "Drugs are not always necessary," Cousins wrote. "Belief in recovery always is."[36]

Is Alternative Medicine Safe?

Like Norman Cousins, many of us are not that concerned whether it is an alternative treatment itself or our belief in it that makes us feel better. But understandably we are worried about potential harm. The most serious criticism leveled at alternative care is that patients who use it will miss out on effective medical treatment. "For some people, alternative therapies could be deadly because they are not getting the care they need," Dr. Jill Buyon says. "Someone whose kidneys are dying from lupus nephritis [inflammation of the kidneys] is not likely to be helped by herbal remedies, and a patient really has to understand that when he or she makes the decision not to go with traditional therapies."

Most people who have serious health problems do not rely on alternative medicine alone, according to Dr. Eisenberg's research. He found that unconventional therapies generally are used as an adjunct to, rather than as a replacement for, conventional medicine. Among respondents who used unconventional medicine to treat their principal medical condition in both 1991 and 1997, only 4 percent saw an alternative practitioner without also seeing a medical doctor.[37]

Another concern about alternative care is its costs. "The major side effect of alternative medicine is poverty," my doctor used to tell me. Though most of us have medical insurance and some level of prescription drug coverage, we pay the lion's share of alternative care—more than $10 billion worth in 1990—out of our own pockets. Licensed massage therapist Virginia Touhey of Clifton Park, New York, laments the fact that for many of her clients, insurance will cover the knife, but it won't cover massage. For many of us, the expense of alternative care puts it beyond our reach.

Mireille, for example, receives disability payments for a back injury and fibromyalgia. She tried an herbal remedy recommended for its ability to fight fatigue, but she couldn't afford to buy a therapeutic dosage. She felt chiropractic lessened her pain, but her health insurance covered a limited number of visits and paid only part of the cost. Acupuncture also was too expensive. "My pension is enough to live on, but it isn't enough to add on all these extra costs," Mireille says. She enrolled in tai chi classes, a Chinese system of meditative exercises, and she is learning relaxation techniques.

Off-Label Use of Drugs.   If we can afford alternative care, and we are not using it to avoid needed medical treatment, what is the harm? Critics point to some potentially serious, and even deadly, side effects of certain unconventional treatments. While I was researching this book, one of the most hotly debated treatments for fibromyalgia and chronic fatigue syndrome was the so-called off-label use of the diet drugs fenfluramine and phentermine, taken in combination. An "off-label" use refers to the use of a drug for purposes other than that for which it was developed. Physicians legally may prescribe any drug approved by the FDA for an off-label use at their discretion.

Fenfluramine (brand name Pondimin®) and phentermine (brand name Fastin®) were approved by the FDA in the 1970s to treat morbid obesity. The combination of the drugs, commonly referred to as fen/phen, has not been approved by the FDA, but physicians who prescribe the drugs together do so, according to one account, because the health risks of obesity may outweigh the risks of the drugs.[38] The use of fen/phen to treat the pain and fatigue of such illnesses as fibromyalgia and chronic fatigue syndrome is based on the action of the drugs on the neurotransmitters serotonin and dopamine. Fenfluramine increases brain levels of serotonin, which promotes feelings of well-being and sleep, and phentermine increases brain levels of dopamine, which increases alertness and decreases compulsive behavior.

However, in July 1997 Mayo Clinic researchers cautioned physicians that the fen/phen combination may cause heart valve damage.[39] Subsequent tests by the FDA revealed that nearly one third of individuals taking the fen/phen combination had damaged heart valves, even though they had no symptoms.[40] This compares to less than 1 percent of people in the general population with a similar condition. Most of the valves leaked blood, a condition that, over time, can enlarge and weaken the heart. In response to these concerns, the FDA asked the manufacturer of fenfluramine to withdraw the product, and the company did so voluntarily. According to the FDA, phentermine appears safe when taken by itself.

Alternative treatments that are said to "detoxify" the body, such as coffee enemas and chelation therapy, also have critics concerned. Both reportedly have led to deaths.[41] Chelation therapy involves intravenous injection of EDTA, a synthetic amino acid, which is believed to bind with toxic metals in the blood and cause them to be excreted by the kidneys. EDTA is approved by the FDA for use in treating lead poisoning. Promoters say that chelation therapy is an effective treatment for heart disease, cancer, and Parkinson's disease, among other ailments, but lack of standardized research and the potential for serious side effects, including kidney failure, leave scientists unconvinced.

Herbs and Supplements. To many people, herbal remedies and vitamin and mineral supplements seem more innocuous. We take melatonin to help us sleep, echinacea to ward off colds, and ginko biloba to rejuvenate our memory. Americans spend some $6 billion annually on nutritional supplements alone.[42] Many of these products are available by mail, in health food stores, and through multi-level marketing programs in which customers sell the products they use. I even picked up a small book on herbal remedies at my supermarket checkout counter. Proponents say that herbs have been used as medicinal remedies for thousands of years and point to the fact that many modern drugs are derived from these substances.

Often, the criticism of herbs and dietary supplements revolves around some highly publicized tragedies. The *Newsweek* cover story of May 6, 1996, chronicled the death of a college student from a supplement promoted as a safe and legal stimulant. The product's main ingredient, ephedra, also known as *ma huang,* is a plant that has been used for two thousand years by Chinese physicians to treat upper-respiratory problems. In recent years, the herb has been promoted as a safe way to control weight and boost energy. According to *Newsweek,* the FDA has received some four hundred reports of adverse reactions resulting from chronic use or overdose of ephedra, including "liver failure, elevated blood pressure, palpitations, strokes, and approximately fifteen deaths."[43]

However, even Dr. Stephen Barrett acknowledges that some herbs may have a place in medical treatment, though he feels they have not been studied adequately. He is less generous about the use of vitamins. Dr. Barrett disputes the popular notion that stress robs the body of essential nutrients and believes that most of us are wasting our money on vitamins. Others disagree. "In fact, we have little reason to be so sure of our nutritional ground," says Dr. James Gordon.[44] Confusion in my own mind about which herbs or vitamins to take and in what amounts, more than a sense that they are inherently dangerous, keeps me on the sidelines of this debate for now. As we'll see later in this chapter, we may want to find an alternative practitioner with experience using various herbs and supplements to help guide our choices.

Lack of Regulation.   There is little to fear from taking a daily multivitamin, but many people worry about the fact that herbal remedies and dietary supplements are unregulated. In 1994, Congress passed the Dietary Supplement Health and Education Act, which classified vitamins, minerals, and herbs as food supplements rather than drugs and effectively reduced the FDA's control over them. Manufacturers can't make explicit health claims on a product's label, but the FDA cannot restrict sales of such remedies unless it can show that the ingredients are dangerous.[45]

Those of us who use supplements and herbs should proceed with caution, according to Dr. Daniel Clauw. "People take these supplements like they are water," he told me. "If you are taking a supplement because you want to improve a symptom or make yourself feel better, you have to consider that a drug." When individuals know the industry is unregulated, and they choose to use such products anyway, Dr. Clauw says, "It's a case of 'let the buyer beware.'"

A cautionary tale of particular significance to those of us with such illnesses as fibromyalgia and chronic fatigue syndrome is the 1990 FDA recall of L-tryptophan, an amino acid that is a precursor of the brain chemical serotonin. Many of us, myself included, took this supplement, which was widely available in health food stores, to promote restful sleep and decrease pain. In fact my doctor recommended it to me, with the caveat that he had no idea whether or not it would work. I seemed to sleep more soundly when I took it, without the morning-after grogginess of many of the antidepressants I had tried.

However, a number of people who were taking L-tryptophan became ill with a rare disorder characterized by severe muscle pain and an increase in eosinophils, a type of white blood cell. The Centers for Disease Control, which called the illness eosinophilia myalgia syndrome (EMS), reported thirty-eight deaths from complications of EMS through July 1992.[46] Though the problem eventually was traced to a single Japanese firm, which is believed to have introduced a contaminant into the product when it changed its manufacturing process, the ban on most forms of L-tryptophan remains.

Despite my earlier stated concerns about supplements, my own positive experience with L-tryptophan leaves no doubt in my mind that I will run down to the health food store in a minute if it becomes widely available again. However, I won't be as complacent about its relative safety. Perhaps this reveals some of my own ambivalence about alternative treatments. Research and cautions aside, the most important deciding factor in my mind always will be whether or not a treatment works for me.

Economic and Therapeutic Rivals.   Proponents of herbal remedies and dietary supplements think that a reason other than their potential danger upsets the medical profession. They believe it is equally likely that conventional medicine is wary of these products because they are, in Dr. James Gordon's words, "democratic tools for health" that are seen as "therapeutic and economic rivals."[47] Miryam Williamson is more blunt in her assessment. She finds relief for many of her fibromyalgia symptoms from 5-hydroxytryptophan, or 5-htp, a breakdown product of L-tryptophan that is legally available from several sources in the United States. "People who listen to the argument that these products can be dangerous are listening to drug company propaganda," she told me. "We're never going to see the kinds of tests on food supplements that we see on drugs because nobody has an investment in selling them." Dr. Gordon notes that pharmaceutical companies spend significant amounts studying drugs on which they will hold a patent for seventeen years.

WHAT'S A POOR PERSON TO DO?

We're told to be cautious about alternative treatments but also to be skeptical that conventional medicine holds much hope for the treatment of chronic disease. Daily, we're buffeted with news of miracle cures that eventually are revealed to be ineffective or dangerous. Family members, friends, and even total strangers offer us advice. As one of the individuals I interviewed asked me, "What's a poor person to do?" The answer is simpler than I imagined. Whether we cling to conventional or alternative medicine, or espouse a blend of both, we choose those methods that are right for us. This is not a cop-out but a reasoned decision that reflects our values, our comfort level with trying new things, and our knowledge about our bodies and our diseases.

Know Yourself

Jeri depends on a blend of alternative therapies, including homeopathy, meditation, imagery, and the use of humor to keep her lupus symptoms at bay. Still, she considers herself to be somewhat traditional, and she visits conventional doctors when the need arises. "I'm not going to chase after every alternative therapy," she says. "I'm going to be aware of what resounds in me." Like Jeri, I'm more likely to try a product or service that sounds good to me at a gut level. Going on instinct alone, I rejected the idea of using bee venom, delivered by injection or through the use of live honey bees, which is thought by some to be a remedy for arthritis and other inflammatory and degenerative diseases. I couldn't overcome a lifelong fear of bees even if my arthritis improved!

To judge the appropriateness of an alternative treatment, Sally relies on three factors. The first is the likelihood that a remedy will produce negative side effects. Next, she looks for any studies that have been done on the treatment or product. Finally, she evaluates what she calls the inconvenience factor—how much it will cost or hurt to take it. She says, "If something's cheap, easy to obtain, and there's very little chance of harmful side effects, I'm more likely to try it." Based on this method, she was willing to try Evening Primrose oil, an extract of the Evening Primrose plant often used to fight fatigue and lessen premenstrual symptoms.

Beware of Miracle Cures

Another concern about alternative medicine that many of us share is whether or not a person promoting a product has any financial interest in it. A provider who sells his own prescriptions or treatment regimen ought to raise a red flag in our minds, because treatments that may truly benefit patients with a particular disease are widely available and not the province of a few providers. Many of us also are wary about a doctor's alleged success rate, particularly for an illness like chronic fatigue syndrome that has no definitive, biological markers. "When a doctor says that 80 percent of his patients get better, it's just not true," Sally says, "because if it were, everybody would be seeing this doctor, and we'd all be better."

Weigh Advice Carefully

Many of us are skeptical about the advice we receive from well-meaning friends. No one ever suggested I get stung by bees, but I have been advised to stop eating the so-called nightshade vegetables, such as potatoes and tomatoes, and to have all my dental fillings removed. Even when such practices seem to help others, I'm reluctant to try anything that doesn't feel right to me. In chapter 7, we'll examine the question of how to handle unsolicited advice gracefully.

We should be even more careful about the advice of strangers. Internet discussion groups provide valuable benefits, including the chance to share insights and support with people who have similar problems. But the unregulated nature of the medium leaves us open to being barraged with news of the latest "miracle cure." I even recall hearing about a woman who claimed her multiple sclerosis was cured when she was hit by lightning. Few recommended treatments are that drastic. Indeed, most of us agree that we don't mind hearing what others have tried, but we draw the line at being told that they have found *the* answer.

Typically, Internet flame wars begin when somebody insists that everyone walk the same way, Dulce told me. I love her homespun response. "I say, 'Crabs walk sideways and lobsters walk straight, but they both get where they're going.'"

Treat Serious Symptoms Seriously

In the course of our disease, many of us must rely on conventional remedies to treat our more serious symptoms. Bob didn't hesitate to take prednisone to control his Crohn's disease because he knew that left unchecked, his illness might lead to the loss of part or all of his colon. But many of us with chronic disease end up relying on both conventional medicine and alternative care in our continuing search to feel better. Often, we use alternative medicine to help us cope with our ongoing symptoms and conventional medicine to remedy acute exacerbations. Now that his illness is safely under control, Bob focuses on further improving his health by exercising and watching what he eats.

Likewise, Wendy Hay injects medication every other day to reduce flare-ups of her multiple sclerosis but she also takes bilberry extract, a supplement first used during World War II to improve the vision of British pilots flying night missions. "I haven't had any more problems with my vision," Wendy says, "but who knows if this is just a remission. I figure I'll keep on taking it because it's not hurting me." Before deciding to try bilberry, she conducted a thorough review of available research, being careful to avoid the endorsements of commercial firms that wanted to sell her the product.

Find a Reliable Guide

Relying on our own judgment when choosing an alternative treatment is a wise place to start. But, just as we would with conventional medicine, it's also a good idea to find someone to guide our efforts. We need to know enough about our disease and our temperament to find a provider with whom we'll feel comfortable.

Many of the individuals I interviewed agree that we should choose as our guide to alternative care a licensed physician, either a medical doctor or a doctor of osteopathy, who practices some alternative techniques or can refer us to providers who do. At the very least, Dr. Gordon told me, we should expect our physicians to have an opinion on alternative therapies. "Doctors who are uncomfortable discussing unconventional treatments should get over it. Physicians should be more concerned about your health than their ideology." In the best of all possible worlds this might be the case, but many of our physicians are reluctant or unwilling to entertain ideas about alternative care. Those of us who want to explore such options are better served to find a doctor with similar leanings than to use alternative therapies behind our physician's back. That way, if we have a negative or unusual reaction to a product or treatment, we have a medical professional to address our concerns.

Evaluate Media Reports

Because much of what we learn about both conventional and alternative medicine comes to us from various media reports, Dr. Timothy McCall offers some tips for helping us make sense of what we read and hear. When evaluating medical reports, he writes, we should look for information that comes from reputable medical journals, that is reported by neutral observers rather than by the study's authors, that is a confirmed rather than a preliminary finding, and that applies to a group of people who are just like us.[48]

SEARCHING FOR QUALITY

To find appropriate treatments for our disease, we first must give up looking for a cure. We don't have to give up *hope* that ongoing research one day will yield the answers we seek. Indeed, hopelessness makes us feel like victims, which is not conducive to healing. But setting aside our search for the magic bullet helps us focus on realistic ways to reclaim some quality in our lives. Finding the delicate balance between the benefits and the side effects of medication, and between conventional and alternative treatments, requires patience, persistence, and an unwavering belief that we have both a right and a responsibility to take charge of our health.

DISCOVERING WHAT
MAKES US FEEL WELL

Healing is a matter of time, but it is sometimes
also a matter of opportunity.
HIPPOCRATES

Managing our health can be a full-time job. Whether we get a massage, meditate, or eat a specially prepared diet, we are constantly in tune with our bodies, watching for signs that what we are doing makes a difference. Figuring out what helps us feel better frequently is a process of trial and error, and a frustrating one at that. Sometimes it's hard to replicate the conditions that lead to a good day, or to predict where a bad day went wrong. I liken this to my experience as a new mother. Just when I figured out how many naps my son would take and how often he would nurse, his schedule changed. I learned to expect the unexpected.

In this chapter, we'll take a look at some of the treatments we try that help us begin to heal. Just as our symptoms are unique, so too is our decision about treatment options. The specific therapies highlighted in these pages are those that were mentioned most often or recommended highly by individuals I interviewed. Not all of these treatments are considered alternative. Exercise and cognitive behavioral therapy, for example, are recommended by many mainstream practitioners to remedy a wide range of complaints.

But each of the treatments we'll discuss has been well researched by the individuals who use them, all have provided a sense of hope and some relief from painful and debilitating conditions, and none seems terribly harmful. Many of these treatments fall into the general category of self-care, those things we learn to do for ourselves to improve our health. Ultimately, living every day with chronic disease demands our thoughtful consideration and our active involvement, behaviors that may themselves help improve our health.

LIKE CURES LIKE: HOMEOPATHY

Of all the alternative treatments we try, homeopathy evokes one of the strongest responses, both positive and negative. Dr. Stephen Barrett, a retired psychiatrist and board member of the National Council Against Health Fraud, calls it "the medical equivalent of insanity," while Lexiann Grant-Snider says she is living proof that homeopathy works. When Lexiann was diagnosed with chronic hepatitis, her doctor told her there was no hope of treatment. "That was unacceptable to me," Lexiann says, "so I researched alternative medicine. I came up with two choices, acupuncture and homeopathy. Not being a fan of needles, I chose homeopathy." Two years after treatment by a physician who practices homeopathy, Lexiann's liver is still inflamed, but she tests negative for hepatitis.

Homeopathy was developed in the early nineteenth century by German physician Samuel Hahnemann. He and his followers viewed disease symptoms as signs that the body was attempting to heal itself. By treating the patient with substances that produced similar disease symptoms in healthy people, he hoped to provoke the body's immune response.[1] In this sense, homeopathic treatment resembles vaccination. This *law of similars*, the belief that "like cures like," is the first of three principles of homeopathy, and it makes sense to Lexiann. "Traditional medicines work against our symptoms by masking and preventing them," she says. "Homeopathic remedies actually invoke the symptoms to clear the body."

Individualized Treatment

The second homeopathic principle is called *the law of the single remedy* and refers to the fact that homeopaths believe there is a single remedy, characteristic of each person, that is sufficient to cure his or her symptoms. To develop a unique treatment, the homeopath must know his or her patient well. This is one of the aspects of homeopathy that Lexiann likes best. "My homeopath doesn't just ask me how my joints feel," Lexiann says. "He asks me if I've had a lot of stress or if I've been depressed. He deals with every possible level of lack of well-being."

Jeri agrees. She sees a doctor who practices homeopathy and helps treat her for lupus. "My doctor doesn't treat symptoms," Jeri says. "He treats *me*." He asks Jeri about her symptoms, but he also asks her what foods she likes to eat and what mood she is in. In this way, Jeri says, "My doctor begins to know more about me and about my disease."

Dilution to Achieve Strength

The third principle of homeopathy, and the one that has become central to its practice, also is the one that has raised the most eyebrows. The *law of infinitesimals* holds that the more dilute a remedy is, the more potent it becomes. In fact, Hahnemann believed "the most potent medications were those that were so dilute that it was highly unlikely that even a single molecule of the original remedy remained in the pill or liquid," notes Dr. James S. Gordon.[2] Homeopathic remedies are prepared by taking one part of a mineral or plant substance, diluting it in nine or ninety-nine parts distilled water, and shaking it vigorously. One part of the resultant solution is diluted in the same manner, and the process is repeated until the desired dilution is achieved.

In a sense, a homeopathic remedy is nothing more than distilled water. Hahnemann believed that an imprint of the substance remained in the solution and was made more potent with each subsequent dilution and shaking. More current theories suggest that the solution contains an electromagnetic charge that activates what Hahnemann called the body's "vital force."

Modern science eschews these explanations, and research results have been inconclusive. A 1991 *British Medical Journal* review of 107 controlled trials found that 81 of the studies seemed to support the effectiveness of homeopathy, though many employed questionable scientific methods. Fifteen of the twenty-three best-designed trials showed that homeopathic remedies were helpful, particularly in relieving the symptoms of fibromyalgia, migraine headaches, hay fever, and diarrhea.[3]

Though he is uncertain about how homeopathy works, Dr. James Gordon says he is also excited about the possibilities of this therapy for the treatment of chronic disease. He points out that homeopathic remedies are inexpensive, easy to use, and completely nontoxic. But California oncologist Wallace I. Sampson feels differently. "Homeopathy enjoyed some success during the nineteenth century when its methods (the equivalent of doing nothing) were less dangerous than some of the other treatments of that period. Today," Dr. Sampson says, "its use is utter nonsense."[4]

Jeri and Lexiann don't think so, yet they offer some caveats for those of us interested in pursuing this route. It was Jeri's brother who suggested she try homeopathy, but she labored over her decision. She was afraid she would be advised to stop taking medication she felt she needed. "I was petrified," Jeri says of her first visit. "My surprise was that the doctor didn't ask me to stop all my medications at once. We began to chip away at them one by one." She recommends that we look for a homeopath who weans patients off medication gradually in order to avoid potentially serious medical problems.

Finding a Homeopath

Both Jeri and Lexiann see homeopaths who are licensed physicians, something they highly recommend. Guidelines vary from state to state for the three thousand practicing homeopaths in this country, who include medical doctors, osteopaths, chiropractors, acupuncturists, dentists, nurse practitioners, physician assistants, certified nurse midwives, and veterinarians. At present, three states—Arizona, Connecticut, and Nevada—license physicians who practice homeopathy. According to the National Center for Homeopathy in Alexandria, Virginia, other licensed health care providers may be allowed to use homeopathy within the scope of their licenses, depending on the laws of the state in which they practice. The center maintains a *Directory of Homeopathic Practitioners* that lists licensed health care providers nationwide who devote at least 25 percent of their practice to homeopathy. For information about how to purchase this guide or search it on the group's Internet site, see the resources section at the end of this book.

If we are interested in homeopathy, we also should be prepared to pay for it. Though health insurance plans and managed care companies are becoming increasingly interested in various forms of alternative care, we pay largely out of pocket for the $250 million a year we spend on homeopathic remedies alone.[5] Lexiann believes that homeopathy actually is less expensive than conventional medicine in the long run because of fewer office visits, fewer diagnostic tests, and lower cost of treatments.

A HEALING HAND: MASSAGE AND
THERAPEUTIC TOUCH

The use of dilute homeopathic remedies to heal may seem like a novel idea, but most of us are well acquainted with the benefits of touch. In high school biology class, we learned that infant rhesus monkeys failed to thrive when deprived of contact with their mothers. Certainly, we don't need research to tell us how good it feels to hug and be hugged.

Massage

Despite such generally accepted knowledge, however, massage was regarded as suspect until quite recently in part because of its massage parlor stigma, acknowledges Tiffany Field, director of the Touch Research Institute at the University of Miami School of Medicine.[6]

Field believes her work is beginning to help massage gain credibility in the medical community. When she published her first paper in 1986 on her work with permature infants, she called her technique *tactile-kinesthetic stimulation*. In 1990, she published replication of her research and called it *massage therapy*. Field's studies indicate that regular massage helps premature infants gain weight. Cocaine-addicted and HIV-infected newborns who are massaged show lower levels of stress.[7] The current popularity of massage is reflected in Dr. David M. Eisenberg's 1997 survey of alternative medicine, in which massage was the third most popular altnerative treatment, after relaxation techniques and herbal medicine.[8]

An Overall Experience.   Those of us who get a regular massage to help with everything from muscle aches to stress know that it works. I was introduced to massage about ten years ago when a colleague of mine, who was a licensed massage therapist, suggested it might help the aches and pains of fibromyalgia. Several of our co-workers were regular clients of hers, and that seemed like a good recommendation to me. I plunged right in, starting with an hour-long Swedish massage, which involved strokes of varying length and intensity on all the major muscles in my body (some of which I never knew I had). Afterward, I actually felt more achy and a bit nauseated. My therapist advised me this was because she had released toxins that weren't able to flow freely through knotted muscles, and she urged me to drink a lot of water. Though the notion that massage flushes toxins from the body is disputed by the scientific community, I definitely felt that the therapist had stimulated my system in some way.

After any initial discomfort, I found that I slept soundly that night. I had less pain and more energy for days afterward, and I suspect the massage even improved my bowel function. In addition, there was something about the overall experience, including the scented oils, the soft music, and the caring touch of the therapist's experienced hands, that drew me back. In recent years, I have begun getting a massage as often as I can afford to. I know that it releases knots in my muscles, particularly in my neck and upper back. But I think it's equally likely that massage improves both my mood and my health because it represents an active decision on my part to do something that helps me feel better.

Virginia Touhey, a licensed massage therapist in Clifton Park, New York, agrees with my assessment. "I tell my clients I do not fix them. They allow themselves to heal," she says. She thinks part of the appeal of massage is that she listens to her clients and gives them the time of day. In addition to Swedish massage, Touhey practices shiatsu, an Oriental technique that attempts to balance energy channels within the body, and reflexology, a type of zone therapy that focuses on the feet. Touhey says, "The idea behind reflexology is that your whole body is represented in your feet, so you can reach your brain through working your big toe." Other types of zone therapy target the hands or the ears.

Moving into the Mainstream.   Even the most scientifically inclined physicians are loath to find fault with massage. Many do not even consider it out of the mainstream. "Massage isn't really alternative," according to Dr. Richard A. Brown. "In many cases, massage could do what medications can't, but most of my patients can't afford it." I pay $50 for an hour of massage, and that seems to be the going rate in my suburban community. Sometimes the cost is out of my reach, and I have to extend the time between visits. Tiffany Field believes that massage will continue to be considered an alternative practice until insurance companies recognize it as a cost-effective treatment. The premature infants in her study who received daily massage were released from the hospital six days earlier than infants who did not receive this treatment, at a cost savings of $10,000 each.[9] Still, she thinks the only way massage will be reimbursed is if people demand it.

Despite its obvious benefits and limited risks (there are certain circulatory conditions for which massage is not recommended), massage is not for everyone. "You have to be open to it," Virginia Touhey says. Many people are afraid of having their bodies touched. Tiffany Field laments the fact that while the benefits of massage are becoming more widely known, "at the same time, we're afraid of touching kids because of child abuse litigation, or of touching each other, for sexual harassment litigations."[10]

Finding a Massage Therapist.   As with homeopaths, state regulations vary regarding licensure for massage therapists. At present, twenty-five states and the District of Columbia regulate massage therapists through licensure, certification, or accreditation, according to the American Massage Therapy Association (AMTA) in Evanston, Illinois. In addition, many local jurisdictions have their own regulations concerning massage. Medical professionals who practice massage, including registered nurses and physical therapists, are not required to have a separate license for massage.

To receive her license in New York State, Virginia Touhey attended a yearlong program with courses in anatomy, physiology, and pathology in addition to clinical work, and she passed a state licensing exam. When I see a new massage therapist, I look for the license, but Touhey thinks that an education, and not the license itself, is what makes the difference. She says, "As far as I'm concerned, what you really need to look for is a diploma."

Information on massage therapy is available from AMTA and from the International Massage Association (IMA) in Washington, D.C. The IMA maintains a Web site on the Internet that allows you to search for member therapists by area code or zip code. See the resources section at the end of this book for information on how to contact these organizations. The agency in your state responsible for medical licensure (e.g., in New York, the State Education Department) may be a good source of information on therapists who are licensed in your local area. Word of mouth also is helpful. Often a satisfied client can lead you to a good massage therapist.

Therapeutic Touch

Therapeutic touch seems to confer some of the same psychological and physiological benefits as massage but, despite its name, its practitioners take a more hands-off approach. Derived from the ancient practice of laying on of hands, therapeutic touch is based on the assumption that there is a universal life energy that sustains all living organisms.[11] Those who practice therapeutic touch believe that disease represents an imbalance in this vital life force. By holding their hands three to five inches from an individual's body, practitioners believe they can assess and balance a patient's energy field. They use long, sweeping motions to "unruffle" energy blockages. Studies of therapeutic touch have shown it to be effective at lowering anxiety, reducing headache pain, and speeding the healing of wounds.

I first was alerted to the possible benefits of therapeutic touch at an interstitial cystitis support group meeting, where one of the women gave a glowing report of how this technique eased her bladder pain. When a feature article in my local newspaper profiled several area practitioners, I decided to give it a try. Therapeutic touch is noninvasive, which meets one of my main requirements for an alternative treatment. Like Lexiann Grant-Snider, I rejected acupuncture, which also is based on the notion of energy channels, because of its use of needles.

Relaxed but Skeptical.   I spent about half an hour talking to the nurse who performed my session, both about my medical history and my interest in this technique, which, I confessed, was partly because of my own health problems and partly because I was writing this book. The rest of the time I lay on a covered table, much like a massage table, with a pillow under my head and soft music playing in a candlelit room. My anxiety about the procedure was reflected in shallow breathing, which slowed as the session progressed. Indeed, by the end of half an hour, I was drifting in and out of sleep. I definitely was relaxed when she finished, perhaps too much so to drive half an hour home.

However, I was as skeptical coming out as I had been going in. I'm not entirely certain why this is, though I suspect it has something to do with the fact that I get the same results from massage, and I don't have to believe in energy fields. Indeed, as relaxed as I was by the technique as a whole, I was troubled by the practitioner's comments about the various energy blockages she said she found in me. Being somewhat practical, I have an easier time understanding knotted muscles than I do obstructed energy fields. The session was a bit less expensive—$40—though shorter in length than my hour massage.

Nontoxic and Noninvasive.   Still, therapeutic touch is completely nontoxic, noninvasive, and relaxing. Proponents say these are some of the reasons for its increasing popularity. Developed in the 1970s by Dolores Krieger, a registered nurse, and therapist Dora Kunz, both professors at New York University, therapeutic touch is now taught in more than eighty U.S. nursing schools.[12] Therapeutic touch practitioners are not required to be licensed or certified; in fact, Kunz believed that the ability to perform therapeutic touch was innate in all human beings.

Like any technique outside mainstream medicine, therapeutic touch has its critics. According to one account, "Some researchers allege therapeutic touch is medical quackery, while others, including some conservative Christians, have labeled it a New Age religious practice inappropriate for use in health care."[13] To those who say the benefits of therapeutic touch are based on nothing more than the placebo effect (the placebo effect is described in chapter 4), proponents point to studies of its success with animals and small children below the age of reason.[14] They note that therapeutic touch is a complement to, not a replacement for, conventional medical, surgical, and psychiatric care. The focus is on promoting healing, rather than on curing a specific disease.

The nurse I saw referred me to Janet Macrae's book, *Therapeutic Touch: A Practical Guide* (see the endnotes for a complete reference). Macrae, a nurse herself, outlines the method in detail not only for other health professionals but for anyone who would like to learn it. Massage therapists, homeopaths, and other alternative practitioners may be able to refer you to people who perform therapeutic touch. Also, check with your local nurses or hospital association to see if health care facilities in your area offer this treatment.

ARE WE WHAT WE EAT? DIET AND SUPPLEMENTS

We are bombarded daily with news of what we should and shouldn't eat. Much of the information is contradictory—what is good for us one day is bad for us the next. A lot of the advice about diet isn't aimed specifically at people who are sick. Rather, it's designed to keep us healthy in the first place. But when we have a particular illness, we may receive some very specific suggestions.

Diet

Nearly all of us who have arthritis have been told at one time or another that we shouldn't eat the so-called nightshade vegetables, which include such common foods as bell peppers, eggplants, potatoes, and toma-toes. For years, my favorite aunt proffered this advice but my arthritis wasn't bad enough for me to want to stop eating potatoes and tomatoes, two of my favorite foods. At least the infamous white-raisin-and-gin treat-ment touted for arthritis sounds as if it might be fun. People with arthritis are supposed to soak the raisins in the gin and then eat the raisins. I've heard it said that we might feel better if we threw out the raisins and drank the gin instead!

According to *Arthritis Today*, the magazine of the national Arthritis Foundation, the so-called nightshade debate began in the 1960s when Rutgers University horticulturist Norman Childs noticed a connection between his own sore joints and having eaten nightshade vegetables.[15] To date, no scientific evidence proves Childs's theory. But that doesn't mean the argument that diet affects arthritis is entirely specious. In re-cent years, scientific studies have shown that omega 3 fatty acids (oils derived from fish) may reduce the symptoms of rheumatoid arthritis. Other research indicates a vegetarian diet may have the same effect.[16] Still, doctors suggest that patients with arthritis are best advised to eat a balanced diet.

Those of us with arthritis aren't the only ones who try to control symptoms through diet. Among the individuals I interviewed, I heard about special diets for interstitial cystitis, multiple sclerosis, and inflam-matory bowel disorder, as well as one designed to help the body work at "peak efficiency." For any particular diet, we can find as many naysayers as believers. Though the link between a diet high in cholesterol and heart disease seems firmly established, the connection between nutrition and any number of other chronic diseases is not well documented. California physician Jeff Kane cautions us not to peg our diets to every news flash. "People promote dozens of diets for a given disease, and are dreaming up 'New! Improved!' ones this very moment," Dr. Kane writes in *Be Sick Well*. "Take them with a grain of salt."[17]

Critics say many fad diets are nutritionally unsound in their overre-liance on, or elimination of, a specific food or food group. The current con-ventional wisdom holds that all of us, sick or not, should emphasize grains, fruits, and vegetables and cut down on fat, sugar, and dairy prod-ucts. The people I interviewed who were trying special diets seemed to be incorporating them into an overall plan for better health. I offer their ex-periences with these eating plans as evidence of the lengths to which we go in our ongoing quest to feel better.

Interstitial Cystitis Elimination Diet.   The diet recommended by the ICA to ease bladder pain is not so much a specific eating plan as it is a list of recommended foods to avoid. These include any number of acidic foods that may irritate the lining of the bladder, such as citrus fruits and juices, tomato and tomato-based products, cranberries, and coffee. Some individuals with interstitial cystitis find that alcohol or carbonated beverages aggravate their symptoms. Foods that bother one individual may not hurt another.

Although some who try this diet are helped tremendously, I've had mixed results. I have noticed that wine seems to make my bladder more tender, but I eat foods with tomato sauce at least once a week, and I drink cranberry juice every morning. Though I don't seem to be bothered by these foods, I would have to eliminate them from my diet altogether and then add them back one at a time, as the ICA suggests, to be really certain whether I'm sensitive to them. Sometimes, we may not feel the effect of a specific food until several days after we've eaten it. Also, because many chronic diseases have natural periods of remission and relapse, it can be difficult to relate improved symptoms to dietary changes. Copies of the interstitial cystitis diet are available from the ICA; see the resources section at the end of this book for the organization's address and telephone number.

Different Approaches for Bowel Disorders.   When Bob was diagnosed with Crohn's disease, his doctor merely told him that if a food bothered him, he should avoid it. Bob took it upon himself to improve his eating habits. "I used to be cavalier about how I treated my stomach," he says. "I would overeat or eat the wrong foods, and I'd pay for it later." Today, he's more conscious of what he puts in his mouth, and more sensitive to the negative reinforcement his body sends him when he's not eating well. Still, Bob admits, it has taken a while to change his eating habits, and he has by no means perfected his style. He says, "I still eat meat, butter, and sweets, sometimes to excess, and I don't eat enough vegetables."

Linda Webb's doctor said nothing about diet or lifestyle changes to treat ulcerative proctitis, but she felt her food choices might be related to her symptoms. The night before Linda and I spoke, she had ordered a copy of *Breaking the Vicious Cycle* by Elaine Gottschall.[18] In her book, Gottschall outlines the Specific Carbohydrate diet, a strict grain-free, lactose-free, and sucrose-free meal plan. The principle behind the diet, Linda says, is that certain carbohydrates, such as fruits and vegetables, leave few by-products of digestion to feed intestinal microbes that are believed to be involved in the development of various intestinal disorders. Linda isn't sure she'll be able to follow the plan, which involves cooking and baking with a specially made, nut-based flour. Linda told me, "It's very hard to follow a special diet when you work outside of the home and travel and you don't cook anyway."

Multiple Sclerosis and Dietary Fat.   When Wendy Hay was diagnosed with multiple sclerosis, her mother bought her a copy of *The Multiple Sclerosis Diet Book* by Dr. Roy L. Swank.[19] Dr. Swank published research in 1952 showing what he believed was a direct correlation between the incidence of multiple sclerosis and the amount of dietary fat consumed in parts of Norway. His diet is a low-fat plan that eliminates all red meat, including the red meat of chicken and turkey, for one year. Followers are allowed to eat red meat after the first year, but on a very limited basis. "Because I've cut out a lot of red meat, I feel less sluggish, since red meat is harder to digest," Wendy says. "I've tried to eat more fresh fruits and vegetables, but once or twice a month I have to have a hamburger." Though she doesn't follow the diet to the letter, Wendy says it gives her a guideline to develop her own eating style.

Eating for Peak Performance.   Mary Ann Lyons, age forty-seven, is trying an eating plan at the opposite end of the spectrum. Prior to being diagnosed with chronic fatigue syndrome, Mary Ann became a vegetarian. A nutritionist she consulted after she became ill told her she wasn't getting enough protein in her diet. Mary Ann decided to try the Zone diet, spelled out in Barry Sears's book *Enter the Zone.*[20] Sears believes that diets high in carbohydrates lead to excess production of the hormone insulin and that insulin, which stores extra glucose as fat, leads to weight gain and diminished energy and athletic performance. Mary Ann is not out to run a marathon but when she started the diet, she says, "I thought I was cured. I could not believe how good I felt." She plans to continue following Sears's plan.

Fasting.   Most physicians, including Dr. James Gordon, recommend that their patients eat a healthy, well-balanced diet. Depending on the individual's particular medical problem, however, Dr. Gordon may suggest an initial period of fasting on a single food. He was introduced to the idea of "mono fasts" by an Indian doctor he consulted for back pain that was unresponsive to conventional medicine. The doctor told him to stop all his medications, take hot baths and then cold showers, and eat nothing but three pineapples a day for a week. Initially skeptical, when his back was 80 to 90 percent better at the end of seven days, Dr. Gordon became a convert to alternative medicine. He writes, "Neither my back, nor my medical practice, nor indeed my view of the world, has been the same since."[21]

A Healthy Attitude.   Dr. Gordon cautions us not to fast unless we do so under medical supervision. He also warns that judgmental attitudes toward food can be as destructive as a poor diet. "It's far better to eat an occasional steak or hot fudge sundae or to drink a potent cup of espresso than it is to pine away for these foods or sneer at those who are happily consuming them," he notes.[22] To Dr. Kane, *how* we eat is as important as what we put in our mouths. "You will generate more healing energy munching candy bars at a pleasant, congenial table than you would slurping oat bran and yogurt from your TV tray while lip-synching sitcom laugh tracks," he says.[23]

Vitamins, Supplements, and Herbs .

Ever since Nobel prize–winning chemist Linus Pauling proclaimed in 1970 that large doses of vitamin C could reduce the number of colds we get, we've been looking for ways to use vitamins and other dietary supplements to ward off disease. In the last chapter, we examined some of the debate surrounding the use of herbs, vitamins, and nutritional supplements to combat the symptoms of chronic illness. Proponents say that herbs are at the root of many medicines, and they caution that synthetic drugs can be toxic. Critics say that herbal remedies should be considered drugs, and they worry that dietary supplements are not held to the same standards of safety and efficacy as the medications that doctors prescribe. In addition, cost may be a factor. One of the women I interviewed pays $120 a month wholesale for the vitamin regimen she swears by.

The controversy doesn't stop us, however, from finding products we feel are relatively safe and that seem to help our symptoms. Several of the individuals I interviewed used vitamin and mineral supplements to combat the pain and fatigue of chronic disease. Many of these items are sold individually, but some are packaged together and promoted as a comprehensive treatment for better health. Often, such products are sold by multilevel marketing companies in which satisfied customers become distributors. Those who find such supplements helpful report increased energy and decreased pain, with few negative side effects. Others have as much trouble tolerating certain vitamins as they do prescription medications. My own stomach seems to be sensitive to much of what I put in it. Also, my natural skepticism gives me pause if I feel that I'm being subjected to a hard sell for any particular treatment program. Still, it's hard to argue with others' success. Because our symptoms are unique, so too are the remedies that will work for each of us.

Many researchers who support the use of supplements still advise us to get the bulk of our vitamins and minerals from foods. They point out that supplements should be used only as an adjunct to, and not a replacement for, a healthy diet.

Sharing Experience and Advice.   There is so much conflicting information about what might be good for us, we can become confused trying to sort through it all. Although choosing what we eat is a very personal decision, often we look to the advice of others in picking dietary supplements and herbal remedies. I first tried L-tryptophan, an essential amino acid that promotes sleep, on my doctor's recommendation. Since the product was recalled by the FDA (see chapter 4 for a more complete explanation), I have become interested in 5-hydroxytryptophan, or 5-htp, a breakdown product of L-tryptophan that is legally available from several sources in the United States. Miryam Williamson swears by 5-htp to help her combat the poor sleep that often accompanies fibromyalgia. Though I have talked to her about his, I've resisted trying it so far because it can be expensive and I'm certain that my health plan will not cover the cost of a dietary supplement. Still, if I do decide to use it, I feel better knowing that I have others with whom I can share my experiences. Many of the individuals I spoke to who use specific herbs do so on the advice of an alternative medical practitioner, such as an acupuncturist, who uses them in his or her practice, or they do their own research using such guides as Varro E. Tyler's book, *Tyler's Honest Herbal.*[24]

Changing or supplementing our diet may or may not help us feel better, and we probably are well advised to check with our doctor before drastically altering the way we eat. But like other treatments we try, choosing our diet gives us a sense that we are taking charge of our illness. Doing so is an important step on the road to better health.

LAUGHING OUR PAIN AWAY

Caught up in the pain and frustration of chronic disease, we may find little humor in life, but most of us would agree that it feels good to laugh. "When I laugh, I don't have pain," says Betsy Jacobson, for whom humor has become an avocation. Jacobson, who believes she was born with fibromyalgia, does stand-up comedy at fibromyalgia conferences. Struggling with cognitive difficulties, she writes all her material down. "I do have a couple of fibromyalgia jokes," she told me when we spoke, "but I don't remember them." We laughed together.

Norman Cousins popularized the idea of using humor to fight pain in his book *Anatomy of an Illness*, which chronicles his recovery from degenerative arthritis of the spine. Watching classic episodes of the television program *Candid Camera* or Marx Brothers movies, he discovered that ten minutes of laughter gave him at least two hours of pain-free sleep. "It has always seemed to me that hearty laughter is a good way to jog internally without having to go outdoors," Cousins wrote.[25] Modern research confirms that laughter produces positive psychological and physiological benefits. Various studies have shown that laughter lessens depression, induces relaxation, strengthens our immune system, and stimulates the release of endorphins, the brain's natural painkillers. People who laugh feel less alienated and more in control of their lives.[26]

Leave it to the scientists, of course, to note that the impact of humor's physiological effects on actual healing have not been confirmed. That doesn't deter Betsy Jacobson, who offers a number of suggestions for adding more humor into our lives. Some of the following material is drawn from Jacobson's paper, "Laughter—A Treatment Modality and a Hell of a Lot of Fun," presented at a Portland, Oregon, fibromyalgia conference in September 1996. To begin with, she recommends that we laugh at almost everything, including "terribly funny" books, movies, and television programs. We should fake a laugh if we need to, she says, since our body won't know the difference. A chuckle isn't enough. "You must be loud and guffaw," Jacobson says. We can say outrageous things and do the unexpected. The possibilities for this are endless, she believes.

Learning to Laugh at Ourselves

Jacobson recommends highly that we laugh at ourselves. As I researched this book, I was struck at how readily the people I interviewed turned their humor inward. Their laughter was contagious; hearing only my side of the conversation, my husband couldn't understand how talking about chronic illness could be so funny. We use humor as a way to connect to others who share similar experiences. There are even books of humor for people with chronic diseases, such as *Laugh at Your Muscles* by Dr. Mark J. Pellegrino, who calls himself a fibromyalgia survivor. One of my favorite entries from this collection is number three in a list of ten ways to know your brain is affected by fibromyalgia: "You avoid salad bars because too many decisions are involved."[27] I've had days that bad.

We also use humor as a defense mechanism. Dulce had cognitive problems long before she knew she had fibromyalgia. As a result, she was known as "the girl with her foot in her mouth." "Everybody thought it was so funny," she told me. "One time I intended to say I was famished, and I said I was ravaged. My form of coping was to turn it into a joke on myself."

I laughed often when talking to Daniel, who sprinkled our talk about his life with multiple sclerosis with liberal doses of dry wit. "Autoimmune diseases favor women," Daniel told me. "I'm in touch with my feminine side." He also made the observation, "I was always a spastic, and now I know why." Daniel says there was a time when he thought, "If I got any funnier, I would die. That was out of despair, but I'm over that stage." Today, his sense of humor helps him maintain perspective.

Lexiann Grant-Snider sends me E-mail messages that never fail to make me smile. In one, she suggested I tell readers that the best way to find a doctor is to "pull their names from multiple, random phone books, stick them on a wall, and throw darts at them. Where they stick is where you start!" As with all humor, what makes our comments so funny is the grain of truth they contain.

Laughter Is Good Medicine

Humor is being taken more seriously by the medical profession. Even as august an authority as the *Journal of the American Medical Association* recommends that medical students and physicians use humor to help relieve patients' stress and improve the doctor–patient relationship.[28] The *Journal* also notes that the study of humor physiology is known as "gelotology," which somehow conjures an image in my mind of what we look like when we engage in a hearty belly laugh. A number of hospitals and health care facilities around the country have instituted humor programs.

We should do the same, advises humor guru Dr. William Fry, professor emeritus of psychiatry at Stanford University. Fry recommends that we figure out what makes us laugh and begin building our own humor library. He suggests that we create a humor corner to house our collection of books, magazines, videos, and the like.[29] Even a few minutes of laughter, he believes, will do us good. Unlike some of the other remedies we try, laughter is completely safe, nontoxic, and fun, with few negative side affects. All we have to lose is a bad mood.

PRAYING FOR STRENGTH AND RELIEF

Few of the people I interviewed expressed a particular religious leaning, but nearly all professed spiritual beliefs. We call on a higher power for strength to handle our illnesses and for relief from our symptoms. Some of us believe very strongly in the power of prayer to heal, while others feel it certainly can't hurt.

A *Time* magazine/CNN poll conducted in June 1996 found that 82 percent of Americans believe in the healing power of prayer, and 64 percent think doctors should pray with patients who request it.[30] Nearly all family physicians (99 percent) surveyed at a national conference in October 1996 said they believe in the ability of religious beliefs to contribute to a patient's healing. Three quarters of the doctors said they believe that praying for someone can aid in medical treatment.[31]

An increasing body of research confirms these beliefs. The majority of more than two hundred studies that touch directly or indirectly on the role of spirituality in healing indicate that faith is good for us.[32] For example, a 1995 study revealed that patients undergoing heart surgery who reported no religious beliefs had three times the death rate of those who drew strength and comfort from their faith. Other studies have shown that people who attend church regularly are less depressed and physically healthier than those who do not. Researchers speculate that churchgoers may have healthier personal habits and greater social support, which might account for some of the difference.

The Power of Prayer

Harvard cardiologist Herbert Benson, who demonstrated that meditation can produce a relaxation response to help combat disease, thinks that faith may have a direct impact on our physiology. In a five-year study of patients using meditation to battle chronic illnesses, *Time* magazine reported, "Benson found that those who claim to feel the intimate presence of a higher power had better health and more rapid recoveries."[33] Dr. Benson speculates that prayer produces the same biochemical changes as meditation, including lowered blood pressure, heart rate, and respiration, and a decreased production of stress-related hormones.

Even intercessory prayer (prayer on behalf of another) has been shown to be beneficial. The 1988 study by cardiologist Randolph Byrd showed that coronary care patients who were prayed for did better than those who received medical care alone. Criticized for certain design flaws, his study has never been replicated.

Lenore's experience with the power of prayer to heal is fairly dramatic, and she doesn't tell it often for fear of criticism and disbelief. "My pain drove me to God," Lenore says. At her wits' end with chronic bladder problems, and unable to afford diagnostic testing or further treatment, she asked a friend to join her in prayer. Since the night she and her friend prayed together over the telephone, Lenore says she has had no further symptoms. She takes bubble baths, eats spicy foods, and has sex with impunity, all things that previously would have aggravated her bladder.

"Maybe this is just a remission," Lenore acknowledges. "I'm open to that possibility. I believe that God's will is perfect and that a *no* answer is as good as a *yes* answer if I really have faith." Lenore considers difficult times to be spiritual gifts, and she thinks her bladder problems have given her a gift of compassion for others who have debilitating disabilities. She doesn't practice a specific religion but advocates the development of what she calls "spiritual muscles."

The Importance of Faith

Science and spirituality make uneasy bedfellows, but each has its place in the treatment of chronic disease, according to Daniel. He is a scientist by training, with a doctorate in physiology and biophysics. He is comfortable with the use of conventional medicine to treat his multiple sclerosis. But Daniel also is an Orthodox Jew, and his father and two brothers are rabbis. He studies his religion faithfully, attending weekly classes with the same rabbi for the past twelve years.

"I am a scientist," Daniel says, "and science is great for a good many things. But it's lacking in any moral values. Science is just a way of describing what it is; it doesn't confer any meaning." Daniel says his faith allows him to believe he is still the same person he always was despite the changes in his body. He no longer drives and has difficulty walking even with the aid of a cane. Daniel's religious beliefs give him an identity and a place in the community, he says, though they don't make it any easier for him to understand why he has multiple sclerosis.

My own faith has grown stronger in recent years, in part because I have nurtured it as a way to help me cope. I never have felt that God chose to impose on me the burdens of chronic illness, yet I have been acutely aware of His presence in helping me accept my limitations and overcome my fears. Returning to church after an absence of more than fifteen years, I came to believe, under the gentle guidance of my pastor, that we live in an imperfect world: even the most faith-filled people have bodies that are passing away. I began to build a community of friends that sustains me to this day and, as a wonderful bonus, I met my husband in church.

We don't have to believe in God, however, to realize the benefits of faith. "I have been on a spiritual path for about six years," Mary Ann Lyons told me. She has learned to summon what she calls spirit guides and ask them for wisdom and advice. Mary Ann likens this to the process of turning things over to a higher power, much like the twelve-step programs modeled after Alcoholics Anonymous. "When my ego can't do it anymore, I have to let the spiritual part of me help." She credits her faith with playing an important role in her ongoing recovery from chronic fatigue syndrome.

A Low-Cost Alternative

Like humor, the role of faith in healing has attracted the attention of the medical community. More than nine hundred participants attended a December 1995 continuing education course called "Spirituality and Healing in Medicine" organized by Dr. Herbert Benson at Harvard Medical School. As with other alternative practices, Dr. Benson believes that insurance companies and HMOs increasingly will become interested in the ability of such techniques as meditation and prayer to reduce the cost of patient care. Still, some doctors worry that reliance on prayer alone may prove dangerous for people with serious diseases.

"Faith does play a part in healing," Lenore says, "but God put wonderful, competent doctors on this earth, and we have to do some legwork.

Getting ourselves to the doctor may be what we need to do." As an adjunct to medical care, however, prayer can't hurt, according to Dr. Sam Benjamin, program director of the Arizona Center for Health and Medicine in Phoenix, a clinic that combines conventional and alternative medicine. Dr. Benjamin sometimes tapes Bible passages to patients' pillows before surgery. He isn't sure whether or not this helps, but if it doesn't, he asks, "What harm does it do?"[34] Also, he notes, faith is free.

RELAXING THROUGH MEDITATION, BIOFEEDBACK, AND IMAGERY

Meditation

Relaxation techniques, including meditation, biofeedback, and imagery, draw on the intimate connection between the mind and the body. Though many people pray when they meditate, even those who don't have specific spiritual beliefs can reap its psychological and physiological benefits, according to Dr. Herbert Benson, who helped make meditation a household word with publication in 1975 of *The Relaxation Response*.[35] He demonstrated that when a person repeats a word, sound, or phrase, often called a *mantra*, and passively disregards intrusive thoughts, a specific set of physiological changes occur. Heart rate, respiration, and brain waves slow down, muscles relax, and the production of stress-related hormones diminishes, thereby countering the fight-or-flight response that has been associated with many diseases. Studies have shown that, as a result, people with insomnia sleep better, women who are infertile can become pregnant, and patients with chronic pain take fewer drugs.[36] Rather than using a mantra, many of us are taught to meditate by focusing on the sound and the sensation of our breathing.

A Time Out.   Meditation is something nearly all of us have tried in one form or another, and many of us use with great success. Meditation provides a "physiological and psychological 'time out,'" according to Dr. James Gordon.[37] It helps to quiet internal chatter that Hindus call "the drunken monkey."[38] When Kathy Hammitt meditates, it takes the focus off Sjogren's syndrome and helps her remember to concentrate on the things and the people that she loves. Kathy says, "When I do this, I don't get depressed." Lenore meditates to be closer to God. Since she and her husband started meditating together, she believes it has enhanced their marriage. Chronic illness causes strain in the best of relationships, as we'll discuss in chapter 7.

"Active" Meditation.   As many times as I have tried various forms of meditation, I always have found it difficult to quiet my mind. That's why I was relieved to learn that there are other ways to achieve the same results. "The practices that most of us associate with the word *meditation,* the silent sitting, the focusing on the sound or breath, the emptying of the mind, are wonderful and wonderfully useful," Dr. James Gordon writes.[39] But the idea that there is only one way to meditate is both arrogant and ignorant, he says. To help his patients who have trouble with more quiet forms of meditation, Dr. Gordon prescribes what he calls *expressive meditations,* such as fast dancing. Massage therapist Virginia Touhey recommends yoga or tai chi to clients who say they can't meditate. Exercise calms your mind by working your body first, she told me.

I'm definitely the type of person who would rather dance than listen to myself breathe. Still, my primary care physician worries that my reluctance to try meditating may reflect an unwillingness to sit with some very uncomfortable feelings, and she may be right. The few times I have tried quiet meditation, I have been acutely aware of negative physical sensations, as well as a wave of emotions about being sick that I don't have to pay attention to when I am busy. Allowing myself to have these feelings, however uncomfortable, is an important step in discovering what will help me heal. We'll take a more detailed look at the role of emotions in chronic disease in chapter 6.

Biofeedback

I had an easier time learning biofeedback, a relaxation technique that required me to use my mind to recognize and alter changes in my autonomic (involuntary) nervous system. In the 1960s, experimental psychologist Neal Miller demonstrated that people could be taught to raise their blood pressure or increase the temperature in their hands when offered some type of perceptible recording of the change, such as use of a high-pitched sound.[40] This ran counter to the prevailing notion that all autonomic responses were outside voluntary control. Miller's work led to the development of biofeedback, which is now used to treat such problems as chronic headaches and bowel and bladder incontinence.

Lenore used biofeedback to learn to relax the muscles in her pelvic floor, an area she clenched involuntarily as a result of childhood sexual abuse. She believes this behavior may have contributed to her cystitis symptoms. "The biofeedback helped me understand where I carried stress in my body," she says.

I participated in a university research study measuring the impact of biofeedback on chronic headaches. The researchers theorized that because people who learn to raise the temperature of their hands are relaxing blood vessels not only in their hands but also in their heads, this technique would be effective for controlling migraine headaches.

For each of twelve sessions, I was wired with electrodes that measured the temperature in my hands and reflected even the smallest change on an electronic graph. When I successfully raised the temperature in my hands, I received the positive reinforcement of seeing longer lines on the graph. The goal of biofeedback is to teach an individual how it feels to achieve the desired result so he or she can replicate it without using any equipment.

One reason patients like biofeedback training, according to NCCAM, is that it gives them a sense of mastery over their illness.[41] Indeed, investigators of the study in which I took part found that control group subjects who were taught to cool their hands, or to stabilize the temperature of their hands, also showed a decrease in vascular headaches. In all groups, those subjects who mastered the technique of biofeedback showed more headache relief than those who were only modestly successful. The researchers speculated that the experience of success with a relevant and credible task may have led to the headache relief.[42] Though the number of headaches I had did not decrease during the study period, their intensity seemed to lessen. I was impressed by the fact that I had far more control over the way I feel than I had imagined.

Visualization and Imagery

Many of us combine meditation and biofeedback with the use of visualization and imagery. Visualization refers to seeing with the mind's eye, while imagery involves all of our senses. I practiced imagery during my biofeedback sessions. When I imagined myself lying on a sunny beach, feeling the warm sun on my skin and hearing the waves lapping at the shore, I could see the temperature of my hands increase as recorded on the electronic graph. To test how much control I had over my autonomic nervous system, the research assistant asked me to reverse the process; when I thought about dipping my hands in ice water and imagined how painful that would be, the lines on the graph got shorter.

Sometimes visualization and imagery can reflect conquest, when we imagine our disease being eradicated by medication or by our own immune system. Other times, it can be more peaceful, when we visualize how we will look and feel when we are well. Jeri chose meditation and imagery over psychotherapy as a way to help her confront the challenge of living with lupus. "I didn't want any long-faced psychiatrist asking me how I was feeling," Jeri says. "Imagery is a very positive thing." It also may have powerful biological consequences, according to Dr. James Gordon. Though there is no direct evidence that imagery can alter the course of a life-threatening illness, a combination of meditation and imagery has been shown to increase the number and activity of immune-enhancing white blood cells in people who have cancer and AIDS.[43]

Learning How to Relax.   Though it may seem paradoxical to suggest that learning how to relax takes work, that is exactly the case. As I learned with biofeedback, we must practice relaxation techniques regularly to achieve their full benefit. Many of these methods are fairly easy to learn, and with the exception of biofeedback, they require little more than an investment of time. Books on the use of meditation and imagery are available in the health section of your local bookstore. Your doctor or therapist may be able to refer you to, or even offer, biofeedback sessions. Yoga centers, massage clinics, and even some health maintenance organizations offer stress management courses that feature many of these techniques. Ultimately, Dr. Jeff Kane notes, "You can't hire someone to relax for you. Nor can you have it done by a machine or a pill. There is no way around your intense personal participation."[44] Like many of the other alternative methods we try, learning relaxation techniques is a way for us to become responsible for how we feel.

MOVING OUR WAY TOWARD BETTER HEALTH

To me, the very word *exercise* conjures up negative memories of high school gym class, where I was the proverbial player-picked-last for every team. In my twenties, I took aerobics classes with perky instructors in form-fitting leotards—very annoying! Even in the privacy of my own home, I feel chastised by video instructors who seem to operate by the old maxim, "No pain, no gain." When we're tired and in pain, and probably out of shape as a result, we'd rather take a nap than take a walk. Yet most practitioners, both conventional and alternative, will tell us we can't afford not to move. Studies show that regular aerobic exercise boosts our immune system, reduces stress, and improves our mood.

Because those of us with such illnesses as fibromyalgia and chronic fatigue syndrome often are deconditioned after months and years of pain and inactivity, Dr. Daniel J. Clauw recommends we begin an exercise program very slowly. "By slowly, I mean start at two or three minutes, four or five times a week the first week," Dr. Clauw says. "Then go up by a minute a week until you've finally reached the point that you're doing twenty minutes of aerobic exercise four or five times a week."

That's how Dulce fit exercise into her personal fibromyalgia treatment program. "I progressed from being able to walk 20 feet a day by literally adding two steps at a time. I walked 20 feet the first week, 22 the next, and so on. Ultimately, I obtained 110 yards, in two stages," Dulce says, "so I know I can improve." For many of us, finding the will to exercise means getting past the pain and the fatigue. Some days, my legs feel so heavy I have to think consciously about putting one of them in front of the other. When I do feel like taking a walk, which is one form of exercise I truly enjoy, I typically overdo it and end up feeling as if I have run a marathon.

"If you exercise and you're in bed for the next three days, you're not going to keep up that kind of regimen," cautions Carol S. Burckhardt, professor of nursing at OHSU and cofounder of the university's fibromyalgia treatment program. Program participants work with an exercise physiologist to learn how to stretch and how to do aerobic conditioning in ways that push them without giving them so much pain they can't keep doing it, Burckhardt says. She advises patients to learn to pay attention to what their bodies are telling them. Part of the problem, I've found, is that often I feel fine in the midst of my walk, only to regret later that I didn't stop sooner. Learning to pace ourselves is a constant struggle for people with chronic disease and one we'll explore further in succeeding chapters.

Exercise Classes

For some of us, taking an exercise class has the added benefit of alleviating the isolation that often accompanies chronic disease. Mireille is often housebound by the pain and fatigue of fibromyalgia. She has been divorced for many years and her children are grown. Living in a climate with cold and snowy winters, a brisk walk is frequently out of the question. Several years ago, she signed up for a class in tai chi, a meditative exercise that is a daily ritual for millions of Chinese people.

With its full name tai chi chuan, "Chinese shadow boxing" is considered a martial art, yet its movements are smooth and flowing, inspired by animals in nature. Research has shown that tai chi helps older people lower their blood pressure and reduce their risk of falling. An Australian study conducted in the early 1990s found that tai chi was as effective as meditation and brisk walking, and more effective than reading, in reducing levels of stress hormones.[45]

Mireille reports a vast improvement in flexibility, coordination, and stamina as a result of her tai chi classes. Equally important to her is that she has some contact with people at least once a week. "I feel that I belong somewhere," she says. In addition to her own classes, Mireille helps with a tai chi class for people who have special needs.

There are very few medical conditions for which exercise is not recommended. Still, the prevailing wisdom applies, particularly for people with chronic disease: check with your doctor before starting a new exercise program. To find a form of exercise that is right for you, you may want to call your local YMCA or YWCA for listings of low-impact aerobic exercise or swimming classes, or borrow a video on yoga or tai chi from your local library. Some patient advocacy organizations have exercise videos tailored to people with the same medical condition you have. Despite having tried and discarded many forms of exercise over the years, I know I would be well served to follow my own advice and get moving!

CHANGING THE WAY WE LOOK AT THE WORLD: COGNITIVE THERAPY

Many treatment programs for fibromyalgia and related disorders also tout the benefits of cognitive behavioral therapy. Developed in the 1950s for the treatment of depression by psychiatrist Aaron T. Beck, founder of the Beck Center for Cognitive Therapy in Philadelphia, cognitive therapy works on the premise that thoughts precede feelings, rather than the other way around. "The moment you have a certain thought and believe it, you will experience an immediate emotional response," says Beck's colleague Dr. David D. Burns. "Your thought actually *creates* the emotion."[46]

Dr. Burns's book *Feeling Good: The New Mood Therapy* chronicles the development and use of this technique. By retraining our thoughts to be less negative and more realistic, Dr. Burns says, we can improve our mood and our physical health. In independent studies, cognitive therapy has been shown to be as effective as medication and traditional psychotherapy in helping people with depression, anxiety disorders, and bulimia.[47]

Challenging Our Self-Talk

Carol Burckhardt refers to this technique as cognitive restructuring or countering a person's self-talk. "We challenge our patients' beliefs about themselves and about their disease. When a patient says, 'My pain is really awful and it's never going to get better,' I say, 'Does this statement really help you feel better? What's an alternative to thinking that?'" In his book, Dr. Burns outlines some common "cognitive distortions" that many of us fall back on out of habit. These include overgeneralization, jumping to conclusions, and one of my personal favorites, all-or-nothing thinking. When I don't feel well on any given day, I find myself thinking I will never be well again. Invariably, my attitude increases my level of stress, and I end up feeling worse. I do have days when I feel fairly well, and it helps me to remember that.

However, when one of my doctors referred me to a four-week class on cognitive therapy sponsored by my HMO, I was uncomfortable about using this approach in relation to chronic physical illness because I felt as if I were being asked to feel good about being sick. In addition, I struggled with the notion that using a behavioral approach confirmed that my problems really were all in my head. As I understood more about the intimate connection between the mind and the body, I realized this distinction is probably a moot point. Further, I learned that how we feel most times is a conscious choice, and I certainly was welcome to feel bad if I wanted to. Seen in this light, feeling bad about something over which I have little control seems like a terrible waste of the limited energy I have. Sally puts it this way, "If I get upset because I want the sky to be purple, the sky will still be blue, and I will be upset on top of that." Having recently completed a doctorate in clinical psychology, Sally uses cognitive techniques to help herself, and her husband, come to grips with the impact chronic fatigue syndrome has on their lives.

Because cognitive therapists don't focus on how a person came to have negative thoughts, this approach is much shorter in duration than psychotherapy. Also, it gives patients tools they can work with on a life-long basis. The resulting cost savings are attractive to managed care providers, who typically don't subsidize long-term therapy.

Dr. Burns's book provides a detailed explanation of the theory and technique behind cognitive therapy, and a trained therapist can help us interpret painful feelings that may arise. Psychiatrists, psychologists, and social workers are among the professionals trained in the techniques of cognitive therapy. The Beck Institute, listed in the resources section at the end of this book, can refer you to a trained therapist in your area.

PICTURING OURSELVES WELL: ART THERAPY

Most of the treatments I discussed with the people I interviewed were familiar to me, and many of them I'd tried. Mary Ann Lyons introduced me to a therapy for chronic disease that I was not aware of, art therapy. Like cognitive therapy, art therapy is a psychological approach that helps individuals confront emotions about their disease. Mary Ann used a book called *The Picture of Health: Healing Your Life with Art* by Lucia Capacchione.[48] She began drawing and writing about her struggles with chronic fatigue syndrome using her nondominant hand, a technique that Capacchione says allows us to tap into parts of our brain usually associated with intuition and emotional expression.

"The first exercise was so revealing," Mary Ann told me. "She asks you to draw what you want to look like when you're well. I drew it with my left hand, and it's the most amazing picture of me naked, dancing all around." Another exercise suggests drawing your "inner healer" and having a conversation with it to find out what you need to do to take care of yourself. In doing this, Mary Ann discovered that before she became ill she was busy taking care of everyone but herself. Also, she was focusing on her work to the exclusion of her personal life. But probably the most important insight she gained was that her pictures are full of hope. "I didn't get a lot of depressed pictures," Mary Ann says. "I think the most important thing people with chronic disease need is hope."

Psychotherapist Bardi Koodrin of San Bruno, California, who has studied art therapy and used it in her own recovery from fibromyalgia, uses a technique called contour drawing, in which you draw your face while looking at yourself in a mirror. Koodrin says this exercise scared her at first because it revealed how sick she was. She believes art therapy is a nonverbal connection to the subconscious and, as such, can raise some powerful emotions, not only about our disease but also about past events that may have played a role in contributing to our health problems. Because of this, she advises that we take this treatment as seriously as we would a prescription from our doctor. "Never forego medications or procedures you've been using," she says. "Your spirit doesn't care if you take prednisone. Keep open channels with family, friends, support systems, clergy, and teachers. Tell them what you are doing, and share the process."[49]

Koodrin recommends Capacchione's work. In addition, more information is available from the American Art Therapy Association in Mundelien, Illinois, which sets standards for the profession. See the resources section at the end of this book for information about how to reach this group.

CREATING AN INDIVIDUALIZED TREATMENT PLAN

The treatments and techniques we've discussed in this chapter are unique, but they share two common threads. First, any one of these remedies is only part of an overall treatment program that we devise for ourselves. Few of us rely on one modality alone. Daniel uses conventional medicine to treat multiple sclerosis, but he also prays. Jeri swears by homeopathy, but she also meditates and watches reruns of *I Love Lucy*. Mary Ann Lyons has used diet, herbs, meditation, imagery, and art therapy in her quest for better health.

I'm fairly conservative in my approach to treating chronic disease, but I do get a regular massage and I pray often. I also am open to trying certain herbs and supplements, though when I do, I check with my doctor first. Even Lenore, who improved dramatically after a single session of prayer, believes that the biofeedback work she did also played a part in her healing. "It's not black and white," Lenore told me. "It's a little bit of this and a little bit of that." She says this approach reminds her of the days when women used herbs, intuition, and spiritual guidance to help others get well.

Second, and perhaps most important, all of these approaches call on us to take care of ourselves. Homeopaths dispense remedies but they also suggest lifestyle changes. Relaxation techniques require our active participation, as do exercise and cognitive and art therapy. We must make a conscious choice to change our diet or to watch a funny movie. Even getting a massage or a session of therapeutic touch demands that we be involved in researching and selecting these treatments. When we try one or a combination of these approaches, we gain a sense of control over our own health care. More than any specific treatment we try, the ability to achieve a delicate balance between medical advice and self-care is an essential tool that helps us heal.

6

FROM DENIAL TO ACCEPTANCE AND BACK AGAIN

*Acceptance, submission, surrender—whatever one chooses to call
it, this mental shift may be the master key that unlocks healing.*[1]
DR. ANDREW WEIL

The most important fact we need to know about the strong emotions that
accompany chronic disease is that everybody has them. At one time or another, we've all felt angry, sad, depressed, frightened, ashamed, or lonely.
By and large, we've learned to manage the physical changes that come with
chronic illness. The more difficult part is knowing how to respond emotionally to something that becomes limiting and that is uncomfortable all the
time, according to Dr. Ernesto Vasquez of Columbus, Ohio, a psychiatrist in
private practice who has fibromyalgia and chronic fatigue syndrome.

In this chapter, we'll discuss some of the normal but painful feelings
that accompany chronic illness. As normal as these feelings may be, they
can disrupt our lives. We'll explore some ways to find the support we
need, in groups, on-line, and through professional therapy.

The results of our self-exploration may be a hard-fought and sometimes tentative acceptance of our lives with chronic disease. As we'll see in
this chapter, this is not a head-in-the-sand approach to some admittedly
difficult problems. But given the choice to feel miserable about being sick

or get on with our lives, most of us have made the very practical decision to move forward.

Finally, because our feelings don't exist in a vacuum, we'll make note throughout this chapter of the role that family and friends, society, and the media play in shaping our assumptions about ourselves and our disease. Internalizing others' expectations, we may be striving to reach impossible goals. We'll discover that we can and must be a little easier on ourselves, a lesson I certainly needed to learn.

MAKING SENSE OF WHAT WE FEEL

The most pervasive feeling we confront is a profound sense of loss. We lose our identities as strong, competent, "can-do" individuals. Some of us lose activities we enjoyed and the friends we did them with. Sadly, we may lose our dreams as well—giving up education, career, and family goals that seem just outside our grasp. In the end, we may feel that we have lost control over our most precious possessions: our bodies and our minds. Many days, they simply do not work the way we want them to.

Confronting Our Losses

Confronting our losses is the first step on the road to better health.

The Loss of Our Identity.   "As it constricts your capabilities, chronic illness does no less than change your self-image and your personality," according to Dr. Jeff Kane, author of *Be Sick Well.* "Whoever you were before the diagnosis has already metaphorically died."[2] How we experience this loss depends on how we identify ourselves.

Lexiann Grant-Snider was very active before she became ill. She skied (both snow and water) and went rock climbing and rappelling. After many years of living with Sjogren's syndrome and hepatitis, Lexiann says, "I began to feel I'd lost everything in my life that mattered, and it wasn't a cataclysmic event. I gave up a little here and a little there until I looked back one day and realized I was completely different." Troubled that she might never ski again, Lexiann has become somewhat philosophical about the changes her illness has wrought. "We may never again be able to count on our health, or on ourselves, as we used to, but we can count, sick or well, on life always changing," she says. For now, she has elevated sleep to an art form. "I search for the fluffiest comforters and thickest pillows I can find."

Sometimes our sense of identity is tied to our work. Ken Henderson lost more than his self-esteem when he lost his job; he forfeited his income and his status, as well. Ken had been the family breadwinner for thirty-two years when he found himself out of a job at age fifty. He was the head mechanic for the local school system's transportation department, but he was asked to resign when he used too many sick days for doctors' appointments. He cashed out his retirement and paid off his home.

"It really takes the spirit out of a man to find himself unemployed, with all of his savings used up for medical bills," Ken says. "I feel old some days." But men are not allowed to show their emotions where Ken comes from. "We're supposed to grit our teeth and go on about our business."

At the age of thirty-three, Kelly feels that she has lost her youth and her vitality. Hers is not so much a loss of who she was, but of who she thought she would become. Kelly has been sick for about ten years, but she wasn't diagnosed with lupus until she was in her early thirties. A combination of steroids and what Kelly calls "emotional eating" have added thirty extra pounds in recent years. "I thought this is how I would look and feel at age fifty-five, not thirty-three," Kelly says. "I can't get down on the floor with my kids like I want to." Because she feels "fat and ugly" at her current weight, she is self-conscious about having sex with her husband, which is yet another loss. We'll look at the impact that chronic illness has on intimate relationships in chapter 7.

For those of us, like myself, whose identity is based on our intellect and on our achievements, the most frightening loss is that of our once sharp and dependable minds. Short-term memory problems and difficulty concentrating plague many of us. On a fairly good day, I may forget a word. On a bad day, I don't even have the ability to describe the word I've forgotten.

"Sometimes I have literally gotten a pencil and paper and drawn a picture because I can see something in my mind but the word won't come," Dulce told me. She handles the pain and fatigue of fibromyalgia better than she does the cognitive problems that accompany it. "I was always very proud of my mind," Dulce says. "Now I can't remember what I said ten minutes ago. I feel tremendous regret that my mind is no longer what it was."

Dulce's comments strike a chord deep within me. Growing up, I prided myself on my educational achievements. I was valedictorian of a large high school class and I graduated with highest honors from college, where I was named to Phi Beta Kappa, the national college honor society. Being able to digest and synthesize complex material quickly stood me in good stead in my chosen career as a journalist. But fatigue, age, and ongoing illness have taken the edge off my intellectual skills, meaning that I have to work harder to achieve the same results. I have been forced in midlife to rethink the image I have always had of myself, which is difficult, though not necessarily bad. As I shed the ability and the need to respond intellectually in all situations, I am beginning to discover a more complete and compassionate person. When you can't always lead with your head, sometimes you have to go with your heart.

An End to Spontaneity.   Because managing chronic illness often requires meticulous planning, we lose the ability to be spontaneous. Even before we leave the house to go to the local grocery store, we may need to know where the bathrooms are and whether or not they are clean enough for us to use. To make our trips less tiring, many of us cluster our errands, making certain that we don't have to backtrack. For example, I like to make right turns only whenever possible, forming a circle of sorts, and when I'm having a difficult time with short-term memory, I list my stops, in order, on a sticky note and attach it to the dashboard of my car. Planning for an evening out or a few days away requires detailed battle plans, including lists of all the things we can't do without—medications, water bottles, doctors' telephone numbers, and incontinence aids, among them.

Ironically, even as we give up the spontaneity in our lives, we also lose the ability to make long-range plans. Jeri always prided herself on being dependable. "If I made an appointment to see you for lunch on Tuesday, I would be there Tuesday at noon," she says. But living with lupus means that she can't plan even a week ahead. She asks friends to let her call them the morning of an event to confirm that she feels well enough to attend. "I'm very leery of making plans and staying connected with people," Jeri says. This adds to her sense of isolation. Those friends who are able to accept Jeri's need to be equivocal are very special indeed.

Embracing Change.   Embracing change helps us confront our losses. But change often brings with it grief and denial. "When life, in the form of another person or an event or an illness, challenges us and our habits or even holds a mirror up to them, we rise to their defense with arguments as skillful as those of the highest-priced lawyers and with the demented passion of a two-year-old in a tantrum," writes Dr. James S. Gordon.[3]

The loss of her health forced Jeri to change her entire way of looking at the world. Disabled from birth, and fitted with an artificial limb at the age of six, Jeri adopted a confident attitude toward life. She attended a regular school, took gym class with the rest of her friends, and, she recalls, "I got away with a little bit as a result, which I found to be an asset." When she was diagnosed with lupus, her first reaction was, "'I'll take care of this.' I had a great admiration for my own ability to overcome circumstances." She soon discovered that lupus is a formidable opponent. "Lupus is not something you overcome," Jeri says. "It's something you learn to live with. You respect it, and you make it respect you." Today, Jeri tries to accept change, rather than attempting to make change happen.

A Model of Chronic Disease.   We're left largely to our own devices when dealing with grief and loss, since there are few models to explain the experience of living with chronic disease. Clinical social worker and trauma specialist Patricia Fennell notes that the five stages of death and dying described by Dr. Elisabeth Kübler-Ross in her classic 1969 work *On Death and Dying*—denial, anger, bargaining, depression, and acceptance—have been generalized to other experiences of grief and loss.[4] The problem for those of us with a chronic disease, Fennell told me, is that we don't die, at least not right away. "The experience of chronicity teaches people with chronic disease that they can struggle through the stages of loss only to have their hard-won acceptance shattered with the onset of yet another relapse cycle."[5]

Fennell has developed a model of chronic disease that acknowledges a non-linear, multiphase progression from the time we become ill to the time we are able to integrate the illness into our lives. The model encompasses four phases of the disease experience in four areas of living—physical, psychological, social, and work.[6] By locating ourselves on this map, Fennell believes, we can validate our experiences and reduce some of the fear and anxiety we feel about being sick.

In the psychological domain, which is most relevant to our current discussion, Fennell suggests that we move from the initial trauma of becoming ill—which is marked by denial, shame, isolation, and depression—through stabilization and a reassessment of our values and, finally, to integration.[7] But many of us get stuck at certain points along the continuum. At the very least, we move back and forth between these phases many times during the course of our disease.

Denying Our Disease

Grieving our losses helps us begin to recover our emotional health. However, sometimes we fail to negotiate this important step because we deny that we are sick or that we have a right to feel bad about it. Denial allows us to maintain the status quo as long as our health holds out, but it may worsen both our physical symptoms and our emotional stability.

After receiving a diagnosis of chronic fatigue syndrome, Sally completely refused to accept that she had a chronic illness that could not be treated successfully. "For many years, some part of me denied that I actually had chronic fatigue syndrome," she told me. "I would tell you that I did so I believed it intellectually, but at an emotional level, I did not fully accept what the diagnosis meant for me. I went on trying to live like a normal person."

In the beginning of our illness, denial may serve a useful purpose. Dr. Kübler-Ross writes, "Denial functions as a buffer after unexpected shocking news, allows the patient to collect himself, and, with time, mobilize other, less radical defenses."[8] The problem with ongoing denial is that we neglect to take care of ourselves. Self-care is a particularly difficult concept for women who have been socialized to put others' needs before their own, according to clinical social worker Cindy Perlin. "When you're not meeting your own needs, that creates anger and resentment, and some part of you is going to respond to that by getting sick."

"Passing" as Healthy.   Indeed, we are often punished by family, friends, and co-workers for taking appropriate care of ourselves, and we are encouraged to deny that we are sick because society is intolerant of chronic disease, according to Patricia Fennell. The long-term nature of chronic disease disrupts our achievement-oriented culture. "Our culture is assembled around an idealized work ethic under which healthy, productive individuals are valued, but those who are very young, very old, differently abled or infirm are actively devalued," Fennell writes.[9] This causes many of us with chronic disease to try to "pass" as healthy. At best, this may exacerbate our physical symptoms. At worst, Fennell notes, we may drink, take drugs, or become suicidal as the gap between our desires and our abilities widens.

Sally believes she denied her illness, in part, because she had been sick for so long. "I'd felt this way for so many years that I normalized it," she says. "I didn't understand that when other people mentioned having headaches, they didn't have a headache every day for weeks. Or that when people said they were tired, they weren't tired in the same way I was." Sally spent years passing as healthy both with other people and with herself. She says, "I was trying to convince myself that I really was lazy and unmotivated, all the things my family had been accusing me of for many years."

Like Sally, we may have very personal reasons to deny that we are sick. Illness was an integral part of my life when I was growing up. My mother, in particular, was in and out of hospitals when I was very young, and I assumed many of her roles at home. With the black-and-white thinking of a child, I learned to equate sickness with sacrifice (my own) and weakness, because my mother wasn't able to do what other mothers did. Acknowledging my own illness meant that I saw myself as weak too.

When the rigid standards to which we hold ourselves are magnified by cultural expectations, we have a recipe for disaster. I tried to pass as healthy at work, living up to a standard I could no longer meet. When I sought a reduction in my working hours, my supervisor was surprised. She didn't realize I was that sick because I hadn't let anybody know. I paid for my deception with my health, both physical and emotional. I became increasingly ill over a period of many months, and I was afraid that someone might discover my ruse and decide that I wasn't up to the job. As a single parent, I needed the income and benefits the job provided. My decision to become self-employed, despite the obvious financial risks, has paid off. I don't have to pretend to feel well when I'm not, and that frees my energy to focus on my work.

Anticipating Relapses.   The tendency of chronic illnesses to relapse and remit also feeds our denial. On a good day, we can pretend we're not sick, but we'll likely pay for it later. Jeri equates this with eating too much pie. "One piece of pie is really delightful, but if I eat too much I'm going to see it on my hips." Jeri says. "In the same way, if I deny that I'm sick and I do too much today, I'm going to have less energy or more pain tomorrow."

Angela knows this cycle well. "I've moved from a wheelchair to a walker to two crutches to a cane and back again about eight times in the sixteen years I've had multiple sclerosis," she told me. "Just when you think you've got it figured out, something else goes wrong. Or something goes away. Then you wake up one morning and it's back." Though the timing of a relapse may or may not be predictable, it is a fact for those of us who live with chronic disease that our illnesses will wax and wane. Angela is realistic about the adaptations she has had to make. "I think there's always a period of grieving and of denial," she told me. "But I cannot afford not to do well. There's still a lot of life out there to be lived, it's just a little more complicated now."

Feeling a Sense of Shame.   We may try to pass as healthy because we feel ashamed to be sick. "One of the emotions that gets stirred up very powerfully and very often with chronic illness is shame," says Dr. Ernesto Vasquez. "It's the sense of being defective. As a man in this country, I need to be 6 feet 4 inches tall, with blond hair and blue eyes, and weigh about 220 pounds. If I'm achy and cranky, I'm not living up to the cultural ideal, and I feel diminished." Patients' sense of shame must be dealt with because it complicates recovery from their physical disease, according to Dr. Vasquez.

When Lenore's chronic bladder problems flared shortly after her twenty-year-old son died in a car accident, Lenore felt her illness was punishment for his death. "On a certain level, I felt that I deserved to be ill," she told me. "I felt worthless and defective. I felt I didn't deserve to be healthy like other people." Through counseling and biofeedback, Lenore learned that she clenches the muscles in her pelvic region when she is under stress, a reaction to the abuse she suffered in early childhood. She now believes this is part of what caused her cystitis symptoms to worsen after her son's death. In addition, she learned to identify what she calls a "shame attack"—those situations that cause her to feel worthless.

Confronting the Cultural Ideal.   Lenore's reasons for feeling shame about her illness are very personal, but she is not alone. Patricia Fennell writes about what she calls a "cultural intolerance of ambiguity," which makes it difficult for society to accept many diseases, like chronic fatigue syndrome and fibromyalgia, for which the cause is unknown. People view those of us with such illnesses with suspicion, and we begin to feel a sense of shame.

I think it's quite telling that my husband never realized I had fibromyalgia until six months after we were married. He was aware that I had Sjogren's syndrome and interstitial cystitis, but I was too embarrassed to try to explain fibromyalgia to him. I knew it carried the stigma of being an illness that is not real, and, in some sense, I believed that myself.

Negative messages about an illness and the people who have it are common until a disease becomes integrated into a culture, according to Patricia Fennell; thus, we see terms like *gay plague* applied to AIDS, and *yuppie flu* used to describe chronic fatigue syndrome. Because there still is considerable controversy surrounding the validity of chronic fatigue syndrome as a distinct disease, Fennell says, this condition, and by extension those who suffer from it, are not accepted by society. They may have trouble securing appropriate medical care or disability insurance, not to mention the sympathy of family and friends.

Dr. Ernesto Vasquez believes the same is true of fibromyalgia. He sees special accommodations for people with other diseases, but not for him. "If I am in a wheelchair, there is a ramp for me to go up. If I'm a diabetic, I can request a special diet. Fibromyalgics don't quite belong yet." When we seek the cause of our disease, Dr. Vasquez told me, we really are seeking acceptance.

Isolation and Chronic Disease

We can't share our disease with others. We must live with it, learn from it, and manage it on our own. Because of physical limitations, we literally may be isolated from the people and the activities we enjoy. I find, for example, that the more I try to conserve my limited energy, the smaller my world becomes. Some of the places my son and I once liked to visit, such as museums and amusement parks, are impossible for me to manage on my own anymore. Those of us whose mobility is limited by our disease, or by the use of such devices as walkers and wheelchairs, may become housebound. But physical isolation is only the tip of the iceberg. As individuals with chronic disease, we sometimes experience a profound and intense loneliness caused by being different from the people around us and from not having the words to explain how we truly feel.

An Unspeakable Problem.   Chronic illness often is indescribable, whether because of the intimate nature of our symptoms or our fears of being considered a hypochondriac or a malingerer. Certainly there are some subjects, such as bladder and bowel disorders, that are taboo to talk about in polite company. But the prohibition extends to pain and suffering in general, Patricia Fennell observes. "We don't want to know about the suffering of people who are traumatized by illness, assault, accident, or war," she says. "Because we have no tolerance for suffering, we have no language or symbols to describe it, and so we avoid discussing it altogether." This further traumatizes the individual, who suffers his or her symptoms alone. Indeed, people may ignore us completely. Sometimes when Angela goes out to dinner in her wheelchair, she told me, "The waiter will ask my husband, 'What does she want to eat?' and he'll be astonished that I can read and make decisions like that on my own. I think one of the things you have to do with a chronic illness, particularly one that has a physical manifestation others can see, is to develop a tough skin."

An Invisible Barrier.   Illness puts barriers between those of us who are sick and the people who care for and about us, according to the late Norman Cousins.[10] This sense of isolation is compounded when our symptoms are largely invisible. You can't tell by looking at me if my joints hurt, my bladder is inflamed, or my eyes are dry. Indeed, on days when I feel my worst, I may try to look my best to cheer myself up. Poet Ogden Nash expresses this well in his poem "We're Fine, Just Fine, or, You'll Be Astonished When I'm Gone, You Rascal, You." Here is a selection:

> Some people slowly acquire a healthy glowing complexion
>   by sitting for weeks on a beach surrounded by surfers
>   and seagulls,
> And others acquire it rapidly by downing a couple of hefty
>   Chivas Regulls,
> But whether a healthy glowing complexion is acquired
>   openly or by stealth,
> It's not always an indication of health.
> Your life expectancy may be minus,
> You are a seething mass of symptoms, from astragalus to
>   sinus,
> But if you have a healthy glowing complexion your friends
>   cannot hold their congratulations in abeyance;
> They lose no opportunity to inform you that you are in the
>   pink, when you are as far from the pink as something
>   summoned up by a seance.
> Truly, who needs a physician
> When every friend is a diagnostician?[11]

When I try to explain how I feel, I may have a difficult time helping others understand something they've never experienced. For example, watch a group of women who've given birth share their labor and delivery stories. To those who have never been pregnant, they may appear to be members of a secret society with its own language and customs, and, in a sense, they are. In much the same way, those of us with an invisible chronic illness often feel physically, socially, and emotionally separate from those who are well.

Speaking a Different Language.   For Jeri, the sense of isolation is compounded when people try to empathize with those symptoms that seem familiar. "When I tell someone, I'm tired and they say, 'I'm tired, too,' I feel like we're talking about two different things," Jeri says. "The isolation comes from you telling me you're tired when I have profound fatigue." In Mireille's case, the language barrier is real; everything she knows about fibromyalgia she knows in English, but her family speaks French. She says, "I find myself literally at a loss for words when trying to answer their questions."

Feeling misunderstood is very common for those of us who have some level of cognitive dysfunction, particularly as we approach middle age. People like to tell me that forgetfulness comes with the territory, so I sound as if I'm playing a game of one-upmanship if I try to explain that I not only forgot a telephone number but also forgot what I picked up the telephone to do. I find it difficult to explain that when the "fog" rolls in, I feel, as Miryam Williamson says, as if there is a veil between me and the rest of the world.

This is not to say that those of us who are ill aren't concerned about others or that we want special attention. On the contrary, we try hard not to appear boorish or whiny. "At the same time I'm telling you I'm fatigued, I can hear that you're having trouble with your child," Jeri says. Also, we know that even the most sympathetic people in the world can't truly understand the bone-crushing fatigue Jeri speaks of unless they've experienced it themselves. Still, we want to share how we feel, and all we ask in return is that our friends and family members listen to our concerns. When Jeri says she's not feeling well, she wants to hear in reply, " 'That must be difficult.' I love people who say that," she says. "It's so profound."

The Role of the Media.   Media representations of chronic disease create or enlarge stereotypes, Patricia Fennell believes, and public judgments based on these reports serve to isolate us further. For example, she points out, early characterizations of people with chronic fatigue syndrome as upper-middle-class white women who were greedily trying to 'have it all' heaped social stigma on top of the sufferers' physical symptoms.[12] More recently, Elaine Showalter's book, *Hystories: Hysterical Epidemics and Modern Media*, equates chronic fatigue syndrome with such phenomena as alien abduction, recovered memories, and Satanic ritual abuse.[13] At the other end of the spectrum, journalist Hillary Johnson refers to chronic fatigue syndrome as "AIDS minor" in her book *Osler's Web: Inside the Labyrinth of the Chronic Fatigue Syndrome Epidemic.*[14] Both Showalter and Johnson have their defenders and their detractors, reflecting the often polarized nature of public discourse about chronic disease.

Media coverage of chronic disease tends to be episodic, revolving around the latest research study or the most recent celebrity to confess to a particular illness. People form opinions about what they hear or read that may last long after the story is no longer front-page news. As a journalist, I assiduously defend the right of the media to report the stories they consider newsworthy. But as a person who has to live with chronic disease after the cameras stop rolling, I am uneasy about reporters' attempts to capture our complicated lives in ten-second sound bites.

Paid advertisements are no better. We all have our pet peeves about how health problems are portrayed in advertisements or "infomercials." As a teenager, Bob remembers watching public service announcements on late night television for what is now the Crohn's and Colitis Foundation of America. "I was mystified," Bob says. "The people in the ads had all their limbs and were standing on their own two feet. I decided their disease must be unspeakable." Today, Bob is more forthright about discussing his experience with Crohn's disease with his family, friends, and colleagues. Information on the Crohn's and Colitis Foundation, which is now one of Bob's favorite charities, can be found in the resources section at the end of this book.

I continue to be bothered by use of the phrase "the minor pain of arthritis" in print and broadcast media. How much more realistic it would be to speak about the pain of "minor arthritis." The term *arthritis* encompasses more than two hundred separate diseases. Many of these, such as rheumatoid arthritis, lupus, and Sjogren's syndrome, may involve the body's internal organs and can be seriously disabling or life threatening. This may seem like nitpicking, but if I tell people that Sjogren's is a form of arthritis, I don't want them to think I can just take an over-the-counter painkiller and be able to jog the next morning. That diminishes me and my experiences.

Dealing with Depression

Sometimes the weight of our physical symptoms and the feelings we have about them seem too heavy. We saw in chapter 2 that depression and chronic illness are inextricably linked, and that the question of cause and effect becomes moot. Many of us become depressed because we are physically ill, while for others, depression and another illness coexist and exacerbate each other. The relative physical and emotional isolation of chronic illness may cause us to become depressed, and when we are depressed, we may isolate ourselves from others. Whatever its cause, depression can become a serious illness in and of itself and needs to be included in our overall treatment plan. According to the National Institute of Mental Health, one in ten adults, or more than seventeen million people, experience depression each year, and nearly two thirds do not get the help they need. Yet treatment can alleviate symptoms in more than 80 percent of cases.[15]

During the years she struggled to pin a name on her physical symptoms, Lexiann Grant-Snider experienced crippling bouts of depression. "I would lay in bed, not reading, not watching television, and not sleeping, but just staring at the ceiling," Lexiann told me. "I felt my life was ruined because I'd given up practically everything I loved and nobody had any answers for me. I decided I was just going to lie in bed until I died." Lexiann was hospitalized for treatment of her depression. Antidepressant medication helped her turn the corner, and a twelve-step program modeled after Alcoholics Anonymous keeps her on an even keel. Lexiann hasn't been as severely depressed since she was diagnosed with Sjogren's syndrome and hepatitis.

During the third year of Eileen's search for the cause of her ongoing bladder problems, her mother died. Eileen found herself immobilized with grief and in a great deal of physical pain, and she considered suicide. "I wasn't afraid of dying," she says. "I was afraid to go on living." Therapy and antidepressant medication helped ease her depression, and appropriate treatment for interstitial cystitis reduced her pain to bearable limits.

Wendy Hay had been treated for clinical depression for fourteen years before her diagnosis of multiple sclerosis. "Because of the depression, I had isolated myself," Wendy says. "When I found out that I had multiple sclerosis, it was really hard to reach out and say, 'Hey, I need help.' But I just couldn't do it on my own anymore." Wendy's depression became worse after her diagnosis and again two months later when her mother died suddenly. A local support group for people with multiple sclerosis became her lifeline. We'll talk more about both individual therapy and group support later in this chapter.

Sometimes we try very hard not to feel depressed. Kelly told me, "Sometimes I think I am too busy to the point of physical exhaustion, but for me, physical exhaustion is easier than mental depression. When I have idle time, I just get to thinking about things." She owns a retail catalogue store, is involved in the local parent–teacher organization, and volunteers in both of her children's classrooms once a week. Before she became ill with lupus, Kelly liked having something to look forward to each week, even if it was just lunch with a friend. Today, she says, "Keeping something special coming up makes it worth getting up in the morning."

Facing Our Fears

Kelly keeps busy so she doesn't have to worry about the future. None of us knows what tomorrow will bring, but having a chronic illness clouds the picture further. For some of us, our fears seem manageable. Because multiple sclerosis makes him unsteady on his feet, Daniel is afraid of slate walks that get slippery when they are wet. Usually, he can avoid slate walks. But sometimes our fears are all-encompassing. "Since I've been sick, my greatest fear is that I will die without really having lived my life," Lexiann Grant-Snider says. "I fear that I will experience life in minute increments and miss the big picture, or that I will bite off too big a piece and miss the small moments. I think life goes on in the little gaps in between, and I want to get the most out of life that I can."

Our fears can be largely unfounded, and they can be all too real. When I first learned I had arthritis, I was haunted by the fear that I would end up in a wheelchair, unable to care for myself and my son. I didn't know until years later that the type of inflammatory arthritis that may accompany Sjogren's syndrome typically is not disabling or disfiguring. Likewise, the chance of developing lymphoma is small in people with Sjogren's syndrome. According to the Sjogren's Syndrome Foundation, fewer than 5 percent of Sjogren's patients will be diagnosed with this type of cancer that strikes the body's lymph glands. Yet Sjogren's patient Kathy Hammitt's fears of contracting lymphoma have been made real by two earlier scares when doctors thought she did indeed have cancer.

"You would like to think you've found a way to cope with your fears, but I don't think you ever do," Kathy says. "There's never a time I want to leave my family or my children or be incapable of functioning the way I want to function." She would like to let go of the worry that is constantly in the back of her mind and live naively, yet at the same time Kathy believes her experiences with chronic illness have brought her family closer together. "Many people don't get that early nudge to make life count."

Many of us fear that chronic illness will pull our families apart. "The chronic illness that does not stress a marriage is exceptional," Dr. Jeff Kane writes.[16] Women, in particular, who become ill after they marry may find themselves thinking, "He didn't sign on for this." We worry about what will happen to us if our spouses leave, especially if we are no longer able to support ourselves. Those of us who are sick before we marry often try to discourage our potential mates, afraid they will make a commitment they can't sustain. We'll examine the impact of chronic illness on marriage and family life in chapter 7.

THE NEED FOR SUPPORT

Joan O'Brien-Singer told me that if she had to go through chronic disease without support, she would have "checked out" a long time ago. Support groups, either in person or on-line, help relieve our isolation and give voice to our hopes and our fears. Like the pregnant women I mentioned earlier, we find others who have "been there." We can talk openly and honestly and know that we are being understood.

We also might improve our health. Psychiatrist David Spiegel of the Stanford University School of Medicine found that women with breast cancer who participated in therapeutic support groups lived an average of eighteen months longer than those who received medical care only. Dr. Spiegel told *Arthritis Today* magazine, "'When we followed up on the women later, it didn't surprise me to find that attending the groups had helped them emotionally. But I was not prepared to find that attending the groups actually improved the women's physical health.'"[17] He speculates that the intense social support the women received helped them feel less overwhelmed and more in control of their disease, which translated to real physical benefits.

More recent research published in the *Journal of the American Medical Association* reveals that people who have more diverse social ties are less susceptible to the common cold.[18] The study's authors theorize that people with multiple ties to family, friends, work, and community are less depressed and more motivated to take care of themselves.

Face-to-Face Support

In his autobiography *Out of My Life and Thought*, Nobel prize–winning physician Albert Schweitzer said there is a "brotherhood of those who bear the mark of pain."[19] When we meet others who share our pain, we can begin to relax, maybe for the first time since we became ill. Eileen's doctor put her in touch with another patient who has interstitial cystitis. "I cried when I talked to her because somebody finally understood what I was going through," she recalls. Eventually, she helped found a local support group for other interstitial cystitis patients, part of a network of such groups supported by the national Interstitial Cystitis Association. "Once I was able to take an active role in my own health care," Eileen says, "I didn't feel victimized by my disease."

In search of those who know how we truly feel, we may look for a local support group like the one Eileen established. Wendy Hay started attending a multiple sclerosis support group shortly after her diagnosis. "The group is like a family," Wendy told me. "Of course, as in any family, there's always going to be a person or two who gets on your nerves. But I enjoy it because I can talk about my problems and not sound like I'm whining, which is the impression I sometimes give when I talk about my disease with people who don't have it." Also like a family, Wendy's group supports her in other areas of her life as well. When her mother died two months after her diagnosis, Wendy's friends in the group were the first to know.

At any given time, members of a support group will be at different levels of acceptance, but those who are doing well can serve as an inspiration to others, Kathy Hammitt notes. In 1984, she and several other patients founded the first Sjogren's syndrome support group in Washington, D.C., under the auspices of the Sjogren's Syndrome Foundation, established the year before. "One of the best things that ever happened to me was when I met one of the women who helped us form the group," Kathy told me. "She was a little bit older than I was, and she had had Sjogren's syndrome for twenty years. She was married, she had two children, she held down a job, and she was able to make life work. I thought if she could do it, I could, too."

I sense that's how people feel when they call me for information about Sjogren's syndrome. I have been a telephone contact person for the foundation for many years, and I periodically field calls from people who recently have been diagnosed or who suspect they may have this disease. Often, the women and men I talk to are older, and many are more seriously impaired by their disease. Still, they seem to get a lift by talking to someone who is ill and still leading a fairly normal life. Also, telling them my story helps me realize that I am doing better than I give myself credit for.

In fact, the ability to give as well as to receive support is a critical component in helping people deal successfully with chronic disease, according to Dr. David Spiegel. He believes that when people who are ill help each other, they feel less helpless in the face of their own disease and more competent and effective as well.[20] We experience so many losses when we become ill that the chance to add something to our lives by helping others is a welcome change. As an extra bonus, many of us find friendships that extend beyond the boundaries of a support group and enrich all areas of our lives.

"I Want to Quit This Club."   Of course, not all support groups are equally effective, and spending time with others who are sick can be depressing rather than uplifting. When Kathy Hammitt first met a group of people with Sjogren's syndrome and realized that they needed to use eyedrops frequently, she recalls thinking, "I don't want to be like that in five years. I want to quit this club." Today, Kathy doesn't think twice about using eyedrops.

Jeri found the members of the local chapter of the Lupus Foundation of America, which meets two blocks from her house, to be a pretty low-energy group. She changed that when she became president of the chapter. She invited fewer speakers, distributed more information, and focused on what she calls "upbeat, can-do things." "This disease is very livable," Jeri told me. "So instead of everybody saying, 'I have that symptom too, only I have it worse,' it's better when somebody talks about a problem and everybody else says how they handled it."

Finding a Support Group.   There are certain red flags we should look for when choosing a support group. People I spoke with were turned off by groups in which participants were encouraged to be miserable or angry, and those in which people were focused on finding *the* treatment that will cure them. In addition, Dr. David Spiegel cautions us to avoid groups that suggest we "need" the disease psychologically. He says, "We die because we are mortal, not because we are lonely or have the wrong attitude."[21]

My own experience with support groups has been mixed. It's nice to be able to laugh about some pretty unspeakable topics. But invariably I find discussion of different treatments to be of little help, either because I have tried them and they haven't worked or because they seem a little too improbable for me. Ultimately, when we leave a support group session we should feel helped and guided, not attacked and belittled, Dr. Spiegel points out. If we have a negative experience with a support group, we may decide this isn't how we want to spend our already-limited energy or we may shop around until we find a group that meets our needs.

Health-related support groups often are associated with a national patient advocacy group; a good way to locate a local group is to call one of the national organizations listed in the resources section at the end of the book, and ask for the name of a support group leader or contact person in your area.

Twelve–Step Groups.   A support group does not have to deal with chronic illness. For example, I participate when I can in a woman's luncheon group at my church that helps us apply our faith to problems of everyday life, including chronic disease. A number of us have learned important lessons about how to live life better by attending twelve-step groups modeled after Alcoholics Anonymous. Regardless of the specific problems these groups address, all of them advocate surrendering our disease to a higher power and learning to live one day at a time. As we'll see in the following section on acceptance, these attitudes can help promote healing.

Typically, twelve-step groups are strictly self-help, run by members for members with little, if any, professional guidance. There is no cost to attend such a meeting, though many accept donations to purchase refreshments and literature. Often these groups meet in local churches, but they are not affiliated with a particular denomination. If you feel this type of group could be helpful, look in the community news section of your local newspaper for meeting listings, or contact a church near you. Also, check the white pages of your telephone book for a local office of Alcoholics Anonymous.

Psychotherapy and Wellness Groups.   People who are concerned about the unregulated nature of self-help groups may want to try a professionally run psychotherapy or chronic illness group. Dr. David Spiegel believes that such groups, which typically are structured to run a certain number of weeks and limited to a small number of people, provide better-quality support than drop-in groups can.[22] Many of these are run by private therapists or managed care organizations.

Eileen attends a psychosocial wellness group. When she joined, everyone else in the group had cancer, and Eileen had just been diagnosed with interstitial cystitis. "I thought, 'I don't belong here, these people are sick,'" Eileen says. "But everything they said, I felt. Even though our illnesses were different, I could relate to the fear, the anger, and the resentment that comes with having a body you no longer recognize." Today, her group has grown to include members who have such chronic diseases as lupus, Sjogren's syndrome, and Parkinson's disease.

Some health care providers sponsor educational groups for people with chronic illnesses. For example, my HMO runs a six-week course designed to help people with chronic disease learn effective self-care techniques. Ask your doctor or therapist for a recommendation, and check with your health plan's administrative or member services office to find out if you are covered for such treatment.

Support in Cyberspace

In the last decade, the world has become a little smaller for those of us living with chronic disease. At the touch of a few keystrokes and for the price of a local telephone call (in most areas), we can connect to others around the world who have the same illness we do. No matter how rare the disease, there is likely to be a mailing list, newsgroup, or site on the World Wide Web devoted to our condition. We can exchange information, offer support, and find a shoulder to lean on. The possibilities are limited only by our imagination and by our knowledge of the new technology.

Newsgroups, Mailing Lists, and Web Sites.   Though I had used computers for most of my professional life, and even owned one before it was fashionable, I was a neophyte when I first connected to the on-line world in early 1996. The Internet, that vast, worldwide network of computers, seemed somewhat imposing, and I had no idea what I would find once I figured out where I was going. Happily, one of those free disks that were flooding my mailbox made my initial foray rather simple. In no time at all, I found newsgroups—virtual bulletin boards open to anyone who wants to participate—on fibromyalgia, arthritis, and interstitial cystitis. In the resources at the end of this book, I describe how to find these and other groups of interest.

According to *Consumer Reports* magazine, by early 1997 there were more than fifteen thousand newsgroups on the Internet itself, which doesn't include similar groups sponsored by the major commercial on-line services, such as America Online.[23] New groups are added regularly. *Deja News*, a Web site devoted exclusively to newsgroups, reports nearly half a million posts to medically related newsgroups in 1996.[24]

I also discovered a mailing list for people with Sjogren's syndrome. Newsgroups are open to all, and messages are posted publicly. You must subscribe to a mailing list, which is maintained by a list owner, and messages are delivered to you by E-mail. Lists may be public or private; again, see the resources for information on how to find public mailing lists.

In addition to newsgroups and mailing lists, I located home pages for both individuals and organizations on the World Wide Web. The Web, the newest and fastest-growing section of the Internet, is a scattered collection of pages, featuring both text and graphics, developed by individuals, institutions, and commercial firms. You can find everything on these sites from information about patient advocacy groups to facts about drugs your doctor prescribes to stories about an individual's experience with alternative treatments. Most Web pages include links to related sites that can be reached by clicking on highlighted text.

People Just Like Me.   The most wonderful thing I discovered on-line was that there were people out there just like me. I dragged my husband over to the screen one evening to read messages on the fibromyalgia newsgroup under the thread (that is, a group of messages on a specific topic) "Princess and the Pea." Many of us who have fibromyalgia are extraordinarily sensitive to seemingly innocuous stimuli, such as tags in the backs of our shirts or wrinkles in our nightgowns. Often we are derided for being temperamental or thin-skinned. I almost cried when I realized that other people have days when even their hair seems to hurt. I felt as if I was looking in a mirror.

Ken Henderson had a similar experience. Living in a small town in Texas, Ken had few opportunities to meet other people with fibromyalgia, a disease that typically strikes women. When he posted his first message to the fibromyalgia newsgroup, after lurking (reading messages without posting) for several months, he had this to say: "When you say, 'I can't sleep,' I know you. When you say, 'Flare!' I know you. When you say 'I can't remember,' I know you. And when you say, 'I HURT,' I feel like I know you very well."

Free to Be Yourself.   In addition to reducing isolation, especially for those who are housebound by their disease, the anonymity of much of what takes place on-line frees people to be themselves. "Many of the criteria people ordinarily use to form opinions about others—and on which they themselves are judged—disappear on-line," says Lynne Lamberg, writing in *American Medical News,* a publication of the American Medical Association. "Skin color, sex, manner of dress, weight, occupation, speech impediments, use of a wheelchair—none is apparent."[25]

Mireille compares writing on-line to typing a journal. "What comes through is very genuine; it's not glossed over or edited," Mireille says. "People seem much more willing to make themselves vulnerable." Sometimes, what we learn about ourselves in the process can be as therapeutic as the support and insight we receive in return. The Internet opened a new world for Mireille. Snowy weather and fibromyalgia pain often keep her indoors, but her cyberfriends are available at any time of day or night.

Angela says she doesn't know of anyone short of her husband and one set of good friends who would be willing to listen to her whine about life with multiple sclerosis. "I can get on the Internet and complain to high heaven and not worry that I'm going to turn off the people on whom I depend for other kinds of support," Angela told me. "It's a good place to air your grievances. Then you can go about the rest of your life." Angela also likes that she can lend support as well as receive it. "In a sense, it validates the fact that I still can think for myself, and that I can offer some reasonable advice that people actually appreciate."

Flaming and Spamming.   Of course, the lack of barriers on the Internet is not an unalloyed blessing. There is a fair amount of flaming (the Internet equivalent of a nasty argument) that takes place when people are removed from face-to-face contact. Daniel likens this to the way that people yell at other drivers from the safety of their own cars. When the discussion gets heated on-line, Daniel says, "I feel as if these people are intruding into my own living room." Also, Internet support groups are subject to the same problems as in-person groups—there always will be people who just want to complain, who insist you try the treatment that worked for them, or who tell you you couldn't possibly feel as bad as you say you do.

Spamming (sending messages indiscriminately to multiple sites) also is common. Often, spammers have a product or service to sell, and we would be well advised to be wary. "As with any medium, it's easy to find good and bad information," Dr. Tom Ferguson, author of *Health Online,* told *American Health* magazine. "You can't leave your brain at the door."[26] *Consumer Reports* advises us to be skeptical about any people who promise to treat an impossibly long list of diseases, talk about "a new paradigm" for treating disease, or complain too frequently that conventional medicine ignores their insights.[27]

Scrutinizing Information Carefully.   We need to evaluate the medical information we find on-line with the same criteria we apply to recommendations from friends or to televised news of the latest medical breakthrough. In general, the more reputable the group that sponsors the information, the more reliable and accurate it will be. I particularly like the sites maintained by the *Journal of the American Medical Association* and the *New England Journal of Medicine,* because I can read abstracts of research studies reported in the news. You'll find their Web addresses in the resources section at the end of this book. However, there are also Web sites, created by some industrious individuals, that bring together a diverse collection of materials that focus on a particular disease, a specific therapy, or the general topic of chronic illness. Word of mouth from people who participate in newsgroups or mailing lists is a good way to find these sites. Another way is to use one of the popular Internet search engines, such as Yahoo!,® AltaVista,™ or Lycos,® which will find Web pages (sometimes hundreds) based on a keyword you enter, such as *fibromyalgia.* The addresses for these search engines are also listed in the resources.

The Hard Work of Therapy

Sometimes we need more intense or individualized help than a support group can provide. We may seek therapy for help with childhood issues that have an impact on our physical health or we may look for a counselor—a social worker, psychologist, psychiatrist, or pastoral counselor—who deals specifically with chronic disease. Either way, we come away with tools that help us lead healthier lives.

Discovering Ourselves.   Mireille thinks that finding a therapist was the most significant move she made in learning to accept her life with chronic illness. On disability for a back injury and fibromyalgia, she had lost most of her social contacts. Her two children were grown. "I needed somebody to listen to me," Mireille says. "With all the medical hoops I'd been through, I really hadn't felt heard at all." She sought counseling through a religious order, which based its fees on a sliding scale. Her counselor was flexible and nondirective, gently helping Mireille to discover both hidden needs and strengths. She likes the less perfectionistic, more easygoing person she has become as a result. "These days I feel more certain of who I am, and it's easier for me to be compassionate with someone I know than with the stranger whose body I inhabited all those years," she says.

Problem Solving. Few of us today are engaged in long-term psychotherapy with a single provider. Most insurers and managed care organizations will cover only a limited number of sessions. Though some clinicians are concerned about this trend, others believe that short-term work directed at resolving a specific concern can be just as effective, if not more so, than ongoing therapy.[29] This approach may be especially useful to individuals who find that different therapists can help with different problems.

Eileen wasn't sure she belonged in therapy because all that was wrong with her was that she had to use a bathroom frequently. When she realized the extent to which interstitial cystitis had changed her life, Eileen says, "I cried for the next ten weeks." Subsequent therapists Eileen saw helped her confront the loss of her health and examine options for taking care of herself. "Passing as healthy" had taken its toll on Eileen physically and emotionally, and she chose to take early retirement from her job as an elementary school teacher, another transition that ongoing support has helped her manage.

All Therapy Is Not Created Equal.   When people with chronic illness can unburden their anger, fears, and frustrations with impunity, therapy literally can be lifesaving. But all therapy is not created equal. Like Eileen, I have seen a number of different therapists in the past decade, most recently for specific guidance in learning to live well with a chronic disease. Some of the providers I have seen left me feeling confused and upset. One therapist asked me about "secondary gains," in other words, what purpose illness served in my life. I searched my soul to no avail for ways in which I was using chronic illness to escape life's responsibilities or gain sympathy. I rarely seek any special dispensation for being ill; more often than not, I overextend myself for fear of being considered weak or incompetent. As counselors who specialize in treating people with chronic disease, Cindy Perlin and Patricia Fennell are uncomfortable with the concept of secondary gains. Fennell believes this is simply a way to blame the victim of chronic disease. Perlin told me, "I've never seen anyone get anything positive out of being sick. The people I work with are not malingerers."

Examining Thoughts and Behaviors.   Regardless of the type of therapist we see or the specific approach we take, therapy is hard work. Those
counselors who have been the most helpful to me are the ones who have
challenged me to examine and abandon lifelong habits of thought and behavior that simply do not work in the context of having a chronic disease.
I've discovered that I have a difficult time letting go of my perfectionistic
standards, even though some days they literally make me sick. I have had
to acknowledge that I may be burdening my doctors with unrealistic expectations as well. I want them to be trained scientists and caring parents
rolled into one. Therapy can be humbling as well as healing, and some
people simply don't want to engage in this type of self-exploration, according to Dr. Ernesto Vasquez.

"I find that a large number of people don't know much about what
they are feeling," says Dr. Vasquez, who counsels people with chronic disease. "They ask me if medication would help, and I tell them it might, but
I suggest that we need to talk about the frustrations of living with a
chronic illness. But some people just want a prescription."

Prescriptions can help us manage our symptoms, but only we can
learn to live life well with chronic disease. We always have the choice not
to accept our current circumstances but as we'll see in the next section, we
may be hurting no one but ourselves.

UNDERSTANDING ACCEPTANCE

One of the discoveries we make in therapy or through peer support is
that how we respond to our illnesses, more than the illnesses themselves,
may determine both our physical and emotional health. Dr. Jeff Kane
makes this point boldly when he writes, "Cancer (arthritis/lupus/mi-
graines/whatever) never bothered anyone. What bothers people with
cancer, for example, is not the tumor or any disorder of function, but their
own experience of it." Even when our disease cannot be cured, Dr. Kane
believes, we can be healed when we experience serenity in the presence of
our disease.[29]

Whether we come to this level of acceptance with help or on our own,
most of us get there. We may not always feel serene, as Dr. Kane describes,
but we reach at least an uneasy peace with our disease. The best way to il-
lustrate what this kind of acceptance looks and feels like is to define what
it is not, which we'll do in the following sections. There is no single section in this book that is as indispensable to me as the hard-won and gentle

wisdom that follows. When I began writing this text, I was still quite angry about being sick, even though I have lived with health problems for half my life. I thought that accepting myself as a person who is sick was tantamount to admitting that I had failed as a human being. Instead, I discovered that being human means having limitations and flaws, and that as long as I continue trying to pass as healthy, I will never take the steps I need to get well.

Acceptance Isn't Forever

To begin with, acceptance isn't forever. We move between denial and acceptance many times during the course of our disease. "Acceptance is not a final stage, and I'm not ready for it to be," Daniel told me. To Daniel, final acceptance signals the end of life, and he believes that "anything is possible" in the meantime. He has accepted the fact that he never will understand everything about life, including why he has multiple sclerosis.

"I'm not sure we ever fully come to terms with chronic illness once and for all," Lexiann Grant-Snider says. "After eight years of being ill and mostly stuck at home with pain and fatigue, I am just now starting to cope. I have bad days, and I have good days. Sometimes it's bad and good weeks or bad and good hours. I'm just trying to learn to live one day, even one moment, at a time." Lexiann says her goal is to live well with whatever change she is dealt.

Acceptance Isn't about the Future

Lexiann lives for today. Indeed, Dr. Jeff Kane tells us, "Acceptance has nothing to do with the future: it's simply an acknowledgment of the incontrovertible present."[30] To Sally, this means not looking back or ahead, something she has trained herself to do. "If I don't feel well right now, I can't compare that to how I used to feel or how I might feel tomorrow," she explains. "When I focus on the present, I can decide what constructive steps I need to take to make myself feel better right now." This has been a huge stumbling block for me. On a day when cloudy thinking makes it difficult for me to write, I will plod on through, getting little done. The few times I've allowed myself to take a nap, I've been much more productive later in the day. My fear, of course, is that I will need to sleep, rather than work, every day, but that simply is not borne out by the facts. My fears, however, don't always listen to reason.

Acceptance Is Not an Admission of Failure

We not only compare ourselves to past or future performance but also compare ourselves to others. Typically, we come up short. "I was always thinking, 'If other people can do certain things, why can't I?'" Sally says. Her husband would like to buy a house, but they have not been able to do so on his income alone. Sally has struggled to finish her doctorate in psychology, and she fears that chronic fatigue syndrome will prevent her from holding down a full-time job.

Inappropriate comparisons are self-defeating, according to Carol S. Burckhardt, professor of nursing and co-founder of the OHSU fibromyalgia treatment program. "People who feel congruent with their worlds are people who tend to compare themselves to those who are like themselves," Burckhardt told me. "People with fibromyalgia, on the other hand, keep wanting to compare themselves to people who don't have this illness or to what they used to do when they were twenty years old, before they got fibromyalgia. When they do this," Burckhardt says, "they end up thinking, 'I'm not as good, I can't get as much done, there must be something wrong with me.'"

I've heard this likened to comparing our insides with everybody else's outsides. Everyone has limitations—we just can't see them. On the inside I may feel defective and deficient, but on the outside I'm as competent and capable as other people seem to me. Sally and her husband were able to stop comparing themselves to others when they realized that families with chronic disease carry a heavier burden than most. They would still like to buy a house, but they count as a success the strong relationship they've built.

Acceptance Doesn't Mean Giving Up

Accepting our limitations isn't the same as letting our disease take over our lives. Indeed, even if we refer to what we are doing as surrender or submission, acceptance is not about giving up. "When you are sick, surrender does not mean giving up hope of renewed health," says Dr. Andrew Weil. "Rather it means accepting all the circumstances of your life, including present sickness, in order to move beyond them."[31]

When striving for acceptance, we walk a fine line between denying our disease and taking care of ourselves. "I can be stubborn," Mireille says. "I thought that by readjusting my lifestyle, I was giving in to fibromyalgia. I struggled to keep things the way they were, doing as much as I could, and I ended up feeling worse." For Mireille, acceptance means finding activities that promote better health, such as her tai chi classes, and resting when she needs to.

Sally used the analogy of a maze to help me understand acceptance. Getting sick is like hitting a dead end, she explained. The path we expected to take is no longer available. We can try to knock through the wall and become sicker. We can quit, which to Sally is like saying, "I've hit a block so I will passively lie down and go nowhere." Or we can adjust our thinking and find a new path. "Acceptance doesn't mean we're surrendering," Sally says. "It just means we're advancing in a new direction."

Acceptance Is Not Denial

Finally, and most important to me, acceptance doesn't mean sticking our heads in the sand. Many of the people I spoke with when I began researching this book sensed my reluctance to accept myself as a person with chronic disease. They nudged me along by assuring me that acceptance doesn't mean pasting on a smile and denying reality. I abhor platitudes, and I'm a fairly practical person at heart. Angela taught me that acceptance is a very practical way to live.

"I'm just convinced that for me, attitude is everything," Angela says. "I could sit in my wheelchair and tell you how awful my life is and all the challenges that I have living with multiple sclerosis. That takes a lot of time and energy, and my energy is limited. Or, I could spend that time and energy doing what I can to enjoy life." No longer able to hike, Angela drives to a scenic location with a spotting scope to watch animals and birds.

Acceptance saves Angela's energy for what's important to her, and it preserves her relationships with people on whom she depends. "Obviously, you have to worry. You can't always be happy," Angela says. "But I've run into lots of people with multiple sclerosis who are not even as severely impaired as I am who have pretty much given up on life. Their attitude is so negative they turn people off. I can't risk doing that."

Dulce is the type of person who advises that when life hands you lemons in the form of chronic disease, you make lemonade. "You've got to have a positive attitude," she says. "But by positive attitude, I'm not saying, 'Don't worry, be happy.' That's nonsensical, like hiding behind the barn. I mean positive in the sense that something can be done. I can't function twenty-four hours a day, but when I can, I can do something positive with that." Dulce likes to help others, and she does quite a bit of research on the causes and treatments of fibromyalgia to share with those she meets in person and on-line. Still, she has her days. When the pain and fatigue wear her down, she says, she wants to throw the lemons back.

Acceptance Means Adapting to Change

Ultimately, acceptance means adapting, more or less gracefully, to the changes that chronic illness brings. Some of us, like Jeri and Mireille, adopt new ways of looking at the world. Jeri has become far less controlling, Mireille more relaxed. Mireille says, "I'm more concerned with being than with doing," which Dr. Jeff Kane considers a sign of progress. "You might approach a more reasonable self-image if you consider yourself a process instead of a 'thing,'" he writes. "Take Buckminster Fuller's notion seriously: 'I seem to be a verb.'"[32]

For others, adaptation means a change in everyday routines. "The fact that I can't run a marathon doesn't really bother me," Daniel says. "It's the little things, like fumbling to open a box of cereal, that are frustrating." To have a work surface he can reach sitting down, he takes a chair into the kitchen, pulls out a drawer, and puts a cutting board on top. He holds soap in a washcloth to keep from dropping it in the shower, and he never uses white soap in a white tub. Daniel says, "If we use our imaginations, we can do things differently by making minor adjustments."

To many of us, adapting to life with chronic disease means we have to manage our environment, which may make us seem rigid or controlling to others. We need to eat and sleep at regular intervals, limit our time in the sun, and stop before we get tired. The routines we adopt seem onerous at first, but soon they become part of who we are. Unfortunately, our needs may conflict with those of our family and friends, and we may have trouble taking care of ourselves in the workplace. We'll examine some of these concerns in chapters 7 and 8.

SEARCHING FOR THE BALANCED LIFE

We feel depressed, ashamed, and alone when we live with chronic disease, and these feelings are not unique or unexpected. After all, we live in a world that prizes strength, beauty, and material success. Sometimes, we need to find others who understand how we feel—a trusted counselor, an uplifting support group, or an on-line friend.

Ultimately, living life well with a chronic illness means nothing more and nothing less than accepting our own humanity. We live in a broken world, my pastor often says, and for many of us, this brokenness reflects itself in bodies and minds that we can no longer control. But we can determine how we feel about our illness and about ourselves. I know that I can continue to be angry about being sick and deny that I have special needs. At times I have hung onto such negative attitudes defiantly. "Maybe I don't want to relax," I've fired back at people who have suggested that I push myself too hard. But I'm not punishing them with my attitude, I'm only hurting myself.

When we understand our disease not only intellectually but also emotionally, and when we accept our lives as they are today, we have reached what Dr. Ernesto Vasquez calls a state of balance. Achieving this balance, however delicate, is the best coping strategy we have.

HOW TO BE SICK IN A
HEALTHY WORLD

Sickness is not an individual phenomenon. It connotes a complex
web of profound social effects. . . . You might understand it better
if you think of it as a bomb that's gone off in your living room.[1]
DR. JEFF KANE

Chronic illness is a family affair. Everyone whose life touches ours—our
partners, children, parents, siblings, and even our close friends—will be
affected by our disease to a greater or lesser extent. They miss the person
we used to be, and they aren't sure how to help us. With the best of inten-
tions, they may advise us to eat better, exercise more, and get back into the
swing of life. Or worse, they may abandon us emotionally, refusing to acknowledge our struggles, or physically, deciding they can no longer bear
the burden with us.

In this chapter, we'll examine the impact that chronic illness may
have on each of our key relationships, and we'll learn some important
ways to make these connections stronger. We'll also discuss the importance of defining our limits and stating our needs. Finally, we'll discover
that the effort of maintaining our relationships yields worthwhile rewards—we reap stronger marriages, more confident children, lifelong
friendships, and healthier selves.

IN SICKNESS AND IN HEALTH

For those of us in a committed relationship, our spouse or significant other is the most important adult in our lives, and also the one most likely to be threatened by our disease. We share parenting, housework, finances, leisure activities, and dreams of the future. Each of these areas of our lives may be affected by chronic disease. When those of us who are ill can no longer pull our weight, the relationship may suffer.

Declining health has an adverse impact on marital quality, according to sociologists Alan Booth and David R. Johnson. "Changes in financial circumstances, shifts in the division of household labor, declines in marital activities, and the problematic behavior (i.e., moodiness) of the afflicted individual account for much of the health–marital-quality relationship," Booth and Johnson said.[2] Their research was based on a national sample of some thirteen hundred married persons age fifty-five and younger who were studied over a three-year period. The person who is ill reports less of a decline in marital quality than the spouse, who may resent the additional responsibilities the illness imposes on him or her, the researchers noted.

The unhappiness of the well spouse may account, in part, for the fact that divorce rates are exceptionally high in marriages with chronic illness, according to psychologist Linda Welsh, author of *Chronic Illness and the Family*. She writes, "The disastrous toll, and ultimate challenge for any marriage that includes chronic illness, is that the well spouse becomes a secondary victim."[3] Men whose wives are ill, and who are faced with traditional female roles of caregiving, cooking, and cleaning, are more likely to leave, Welsh says. Socialized to care for others, women feel more compelled to stay with their sick husbands. Welsh's husband, Barney, died in 1996 after a fifteen-year battle with kidney disease.

Renegotiating the Relationship Contract

The problem for many couples is that chronic illness violates the terms of what Miryam Williamson calls the "unspoken contract" that exists in every committed relationship.[4] This contract, Miryam notes in her book *Fibromyalgia: A Comprehensive Approach*, spells out the roles and responsibilities each partner agrees to assume. When one partner becomes ill, all bets are off.

Sally has been married to Gary for six years, but they have been a couple since they were eighteen years old. Both are now thirty-one. Neither knew when they were dating that Sally had chronic fatigue syndrome. They assumed, as Sally had since she was younger, that she was just prone to being sick. When she received her diagnosis, Sally says, "Gary was dismayed to find out that I had a chronic, incurable disease. We were engaged at the time, and we had some serious discussions about whether he still wanted to marry me, in large part because I likely would never be able to work full-time." Sally has just completed her doctoral dissertation in clinical psychology but has not felt well enough to work. Gary has admitted his fears that Sally is taking advantage of him by feigning her illness to get out of work.

"Even if you know from experience that this is not the case, it's very hard to get past this insidious tendency to believe that people with chronic fatigue syndrome are malingering," Gary told me. "They have crushing fatigue, they have mind fog, they have sore throats, but most of these symptoms don't appear on a diagnostic test."

To help Gary overcome his fears, Sally suggested he create a balance sheet, listing all the advantages of being sick on one side and the disadvantages on the other. "It came down to the fact that being sick all the time just wouldn't be worth it for her," Gary says. "The only advantage I came up with is that she wouldn't have to work, but there were numerous disadvantages. She would have to keep up an act all the time, and she would get incredibly bored just sitting home in bed. On some level, that helped me understand that she really is sick."

Still, Gary sometimes gets angry about Sally's illness and resents the extra work he has to do. "I'm winning the bread and then coming home and doing the dishes," says Gary, who works full-time editing a technical trade publication. Their plans to buy a house are on hold. Sometimes Gary allows himself to fantasize about what their life would be like if someone found a cure for chronic fatigue syndrome. Since he has never known Sally when she wasn't sick, he can only imagine. However, he says, "There's no one else I've met in thirteen years that I would want to spend my life with."

Role Reversals.   When the husband is the one who is sick, couples may experience role reversals. Ken Henderson was the breadwinner in his family ever since he and his wife married when they were eighteen years old. At the age of fifty, he lost his job, taking too many sick days to visit doctors for fibromyalgia. "My wife is being very supportive," Ken told me. "Sometimes I wonder how she holds up. She leaned on me for all those years and, all of a sudden, I have to lean on her." Ken says if it hadn't been for his wife's support, he would not have gone to the expense and aggravation of trying to pin down a diagnosis. She has walked the floors with him when he was in pain, and rubbed his muscles with ice at his doctor's suggestion. Ken, in turn, discovered how hard she had worked to raise their two children and keep up their home. "I've noticed since I've been home that there's a lot of work in housework," Ken says. Wanting to maintain their roles, Ken eventually found another job. "Now, I'm bringing in the bacon once more."

Confronting Strong Emotions.   Gary's feelings about caring for Sally are not unusual. According to Linda Welsh, "A 1994 survey by the National Family Caregivers Association listed frustration, sadness, love, compassion, and anger—in that order—as the emotions experienced most frequently by caregivers."[5] In many ways, our partners feel the same way we do about being sick. They feel isolated from people who are well, they mourn the loss of their dreams, and they get angry at the restrictions on their time and their freedom. To compound matters, the person who is well may feel guilty for being angry or even for being healthy, Welsh notes.

In turn, those of us who are sick may feel guilty for causing our partner so many problems, and we may become defensive or ambivalent about our need for their care. The more my husband does for me physically, such as grocery shopping and running errands, the more I push him away emotionally. This is confusing and hurtful to him. "I'm happy to be able to provide the physical support you need," my husband tells me, "but I wish you seemed to appreciate it more." I *am* grateful for his help, perhaps more than I can say, because I'm frightened of becoming dependent on him. I worry about what will happen to me if he decides that he doesn't want to be responsible for a sick wife anymore, or if he becomes sick or disabled himself.

My distance, in turn, frightens my husband, who sometimes asks if I still love him. "What kind of a question is that?" I fire back, which does little to reassure him. Our fears feed each other's until we are deadlocked in a vicious circle of hurt and blame. Slowly, we're learning to break this destructive pattern. I try more often to tell him that I appreciate his help, and he acknowledges that my growing dependence must be difficult for me to accept. When all else fails, we find that a loving hug improves our mood.

Dealing with Frustration.   Another sentiment my husband frequently expresses is his frustration that he can't make me well. Often, our spouses expect there should be a clear-cut solution to our difficulties, and they may be upset when we don't even have a name for our disease. That's how Jim Snider felt before his wife, Lexiann Grant-Snider, was diagnosed with Sjogren's syndrome and hepatitis. Jim, age thirty-seven, is an electrical engineer who is used to seeing the world in black and white. "In engineering, something either is or it isn't," Jim told me. "But Lexiann had all these weird symptoms that nobody could figure out. To me, medicine is so wishy-washy. Accepting the uncertainty has been difficult for me."

Other than some food sensitivities that would send her running for the bathroom, Lexiann wasn't sick when she and Jim were dating. She was extremely tired leading up to their 1988 wedding but assumed it was the stress of the preparations. "Within six weeks of our marriage, it became very apparent that I was not going to be well soon," Lexiann recalls. She gave Jim the chance to dissolve their marriage but he said he wanted to honor his commitment. Still, he admits, "It's tough, and to tell somebody it isn't would be a lie."

To Jim, the hardest part is not being able to help Lexiann when she gets depressed. "She gets emotional and moody and snaps at the darnedest things," Jim says. "But there isn't anything that anybody can do for her. It's that sense of powerlessness that I hate." He also gets upset when Lexiann pushes herself too hard and ends up feeling worse. To take the focus off Lexiann's illness, the couple cares for the four dogs that Lexiann considers her children. The two also help rescue abandoned animals and make the rounds of dog shows. Jim says, "That's something we do together that brings love into our lives."

Addressing Financial Woes

Mere mention of the word *money* can send even healthy couples into a tailspin. As individuals, we come to our relationships with often divergent ideas about earning, spending, and saving money. This can make discussing finances difficult in the best of circumstances. When chronic illness strikes, many of us who are just keeping our heads above water begin to sink under the added economic burden. The majority of people I interviewed had some type of health insurance, though many, like Jim Snider, felt their coverage was inadequate to meet their needs. When they were trying to track down a diagnosis for Lexiann, Jim says, it wasn't unusual for them to meet their health insurance deductible by the end of January. Lexiann does freelance writing when she feels well to help bring in extra income.

Out-of-Pocket and Hidden Costs.   Many of us use over-the-counter products, such as artificial tears and incontinence aids, that are not covered by our health plan. We also pay out of pocket for such uncovered services as homeopathy and massage. My husband never ceases to be amazed at how much I can spend in the drugstore. "Without the added income I provide, you'd find a way to spend less on these products," he once snapped. On days when our financial worries don't seem so pressing, however, he acknowledges that if his eyes were as dry as mine, he would consider artificial tears a necessity too. For gift-giving occasions, my husband often buys me an hour of massage. His willingness to acknowledge the necessity to me of what others consider a luxury is the best part of the gift.

There are other, more hidden costs of chronic illness as well. We spend extra money to make ourselves comfortable, which may seem like an extravagance amid all the other bills. For example, the last time my husband, son, and I went to visit my mother in Florida, we flew down and rented a car when we got there. My husband wanted to drive from our home in upstate New York to save money, but I knew I would be in too much pain from spending two or three days cramped in a car to enjoy the trip.

Loss of Income.   By far the most serious financial problem that most of us face is loss of income. Though some people with chronic illness continue to work full-time at demanding, high-paying jobs, many of us reduce our hours, become self-employed, or apply for disability benefits. We'll explore the impact these changes have on our careers and on our self-esteem in chapter 8.

Reduced income and increased expenses can spell trouble. I've been self-employed the past three years, writing about homelessness and health care for the federal government. For the past year, I've devoted much of my time and my energy to writing this book. Self-employment certainly has benefits for those of us with chronic illness, but regular income is not one of them. My husband works two jobs to help keep us afloat. The second job, delivering newspapers seven mornings a week, was supposed to provide for extras, like vacations and new cars. Now it pays for the essentials, and both our cars are a decade old. I feel bad that he has to get up at 4:30 A.M. every morning, and he wishes my income could cover more of our needs. "I feel like I'm in a double bind," my husband has told me, "because I can't solve your health problems, and I can't earn enough money on my own to lift us to where I want us to be."

Lost Dreams.   Discussing financial issues without placing blame is important, but it certainly is not easy. We're dealing not only with the very concrete questions of how the bills get paid but also with the much larger issue of lost dreams. Gary is concerned that Sally's inability to work will jeopardize his hopes of buying a house. He says he's had to learn to be honest with Sally without making her the target of his feelings. "When I'm frustrated at our lack of progress, there is an unthinking tendency to blame Sally, when, in fact, I'm just mad at the situation," Gary says. The higher our expectations, the greater our sense of loss, Linda Welsh believes.[6]

We have expectations for ourselves and for our children. A daughter in college keeps Linda Webb on the job. She works for a national trade association and does quite a bit of traveling, which is difficult to do with a bowel disorder. "I want to leave my job, but I don't want to go into corporate job number six," Linda says. "I want to do some consulting in computers and training. My husband doesn't doubt my ability to be successful, but he knows it takes a while to build up a practice. He's asked my to stay with my company until my daughter graduates from college."

Sex and Chronic Illness

Chronic illness gets in bed with you, Linda Welsh says.[7] Those of us who are ill find that pain, fatigue, and the side effects of medication sometimes make sexual activity uncomfortable or impossible. The ongoing strain of living with chronic illness also takes its toll. Linda Webb's marriage is her second. Both she and her husband are emotionally and physically drained by their financial concerns and by their respective health problems (her husband has a pacemaker). They have little energy left for an intimate relationship.

Recurring cystitis made sex painful for Lenore. Often, she says, the fear of pain rather than pain itself kept her from enjoying sex. "I would be scared to have intercourse because I was afraid it was going to inflame my urethra and bladder," Lenore says. "I would always worry about how I was going to feel during the night, and I would be scared to death when I went to the bathroom in the morning." Aware that they are causing us pain, our partners may pull back as well.

Struggling with Body Image.   The way we feel about ourselves also may affect sexual intimacy. We may think that changes in our body, the result of medication, inactivity, or hormonal imbalances, make us unattractive to our partner. "The more pride you took in your body—the way it looked, the way it obeyed your directions, and the way it brought you pleasure—the harder it is to accept that it is somewhat less than perfect," Miryam Williamson writes.[8] She reminds us, however, that the fact that we have a chronic illness does not make us any less sensual or able to give and receive pleasure.

This has been a major stumbling block for Kelly, who feels "fat and ugly" after gaining thirty pounds in recent years. She attributes the added weight to the steroids she takes to control her lupus symptoms and to her habit of eating to soothe her emotions. "I don't like myself at this weight, and I know my husband doesn't either, even though he will tell me a million times that all he cares about is how I feel," Kelly says. "We were looking at pictures the other day, and he said, 'My gosh, look at how sexy you were.' I don't think he realizes the impact of his words." Because she feels self-conscious, Kelly is less interested in being intimate with her husband.

Some days, I feel uncomfortable in my own skin. Nothing seems to feel right on me—waistbands pinch, tags itch, and collars feel as if they're strangling me. I prefer clothing that is loose and baggy with elastic at the waist, if there is a waist, but it is very difficult to feel attractive in baggy pants and an oversized tunic.

Learning to Be Creative.   To overcome these obstacles to physical intimacy, both partners need to be open about stating their needs and creative in finding ways to meet them. Closeness, rather than performance, should be our goal. Miryam Williamson advises us to try a variety of positions, to make love at the time of day when we are at our best, and to plan an easy day when sex is on the agenda.[9] Scheduling time for sex might seem to take all the spontaneity out of our encounters, but anticipating private time with our partner may be exciting. Also, setting aside "couple time" is a valuable way to ensure that daily life doesn't get in the way of nurturing our most important relationship. Even just hugging and cuddling may produce a powerful physiological response that helps reduce our pain. Finally, at those unexpected times when we find ourselves feeling that sex might be both possible and enjoyable, we can "seize the day" and feel young again!

Our Dating Days

The very idea of dating when we have a chronic illness is enough to make many of us cringe. Part of the problem for those of us who have been married before is that we are dating again in midlife, which is scary in itself. When we have a chronic disease, we have the added stress of deciding how and when to tell the person we are dating about our illness and worrying about what his or her response might be. Sometimes, this can be almost comical.

Certain that once he knew about my health problems the man I was dating would no longer be interested in me, I decided to be very up-front with my future husband. I also was aware that some of my symptoms, such as fatigue, would be hard to hide. So I sat him down and tried the best I could to explain Sjogren's syndrome, assuring him that an autoimmune disease and AIDS, which is an immune system deficiency, are at opposite ends of the spectrum (many of us find that any mention of an immune system problem brings the suspicion of AIDS). When I finished, he broke into a big smile. "Oh, is that all," he said. As long as my disease wasn't contagious, he wasn't worried. Nothing I said about the effect of my health on our lives scared him away, not even a new diagnosis of interstitial cystitis six months before we married. "Your fiancé must be pretty special to take you on with all your problems," someone said to me. My favorite aunt reframed that statement in a positive light. Aunt Sally said, "*You* must be pretty special if he can see past your illnesses and love you for who you are." The truth, of course, is somewhere in between. Now that he is my husband, both he and I work very hard to make this relationship succeed within the constraints that chronic illness imposes.

Our fears about the impact our health problems will have on a relationship are not unfounded. Eileen's steady boyfriend ended their fifteen-year relationship shortly after she received her diagnosis of interstitial cystitis. "He told me he didn't want to be saddled with someone who is chronically ill," Eileen recalls. "I was devastated. He could walk away, but I was stuck with my disease."

Miryam Williamson believes that fibromyalgia played a part in the breakup of her two earlier marriages. She first married in 1956, when she was twenty years old. "In the 1950s, women were supposed to be cheerful, smiling, competent, and good homemakers," Miryam told me. "I wasn't always cheerful and smiling, and I kept house as well as I could but sometimes things had to slide because I was sick." When she began dating her current husband, she told him right away that something was wrong with her and that all she could promise was to do her best.

Caregivers Need Support Too

We need support when we're scared, tired, or lonely, and our caregivers do also. In fact, while we may put together a network of support that includes other people with chronic illness, our spouses may not have an equivalent outlet. They may be jealous of the time we spend with our on-line friends or at support group meetings.

Jim Snider provides a good deal of physical support for his wife, Lexiann Grant-Snider, taking her to doctor appointments and picking up the slack at home. When Jim needs to take care of himself, he escapes by working or by spending time with his hobbies—computers and amateur radio. In the summer, he golfs one night a week. But sometimes when Jim really just has to get out of the house, he goes down the street to visit a friend. "We may not even talk about what's going on," Jim says, "but when I do something with my buddy, that gets me outside of myself."

Gary talks to other caregivers on an electronic mailing list he started for those who are living with someone who has chronic fatigue syndrome or fibromyalgia. Initially, he posted a few messages on a newsgroup for people with chronic fatigue syndrome, and his comments were well received by other caregivers. But he decided that a private mailing list would give spouses and friends the chance to be open without fear of offending the person for whom they care.

Sometimes, however, Gary finds that caregivers don't want to talk about caregiving. "I have a friend at work whose wife has a chronic disease, and we tried to get into a conversation a couple of times," Gary says. "After a couple of tries, I decided there was nothing to talk about. Our wives are ill, we try to help them, and that's that." I suspect this is why my husband doesn't want to participate in Gary's group, even though I recommended it to him. He has often told me that one of the best ways for him to handle my health problems is to reduce them to their essence—that is, Susan's sick—and go on about his business.

Caregiver Support Groups.   But often spouses do want and need to talk to each other. The staff at the OHSU fibromyalgia treatment program realized that while patients were attending support groups, their partners would sit in the waiting room and sometimes talk among themselves.

"We finally decided we would do a support group for family members, and that went over very well," says Carol S. Burckhardt, professor of nursing and a cofounder of the fibromyalgia program. Most of the people in the group were husbands of women with fibromyalgia. "They felt frustrated and helpless, and they loved getting a chance to talk about what it's like living with somebody who has fibromyalgia," Burckhardt says. "They said it helped them understand what their wives were going through."

Two national organizations—the Well Spouse Foundation in New York City and the National Family Caregivers Association in Kensington, Maryland—sponsor support groups and conferences, publish newsletters, and educate politicians, health care professionals, and the public about the needs of well spouses. Further information on these two groups is available in the resources section at the end of this book.

Making Our Lives Together Work

The problems we face as a couple when one of us is ill are tremendous but not insurmountable. How do we make it work? We begin by grieving our losses.

Grieving Our Losses.   The first thing Kathy Hammitt had to do when she was diagnosed with Sjogren's syndrome was to mourn her losses, and to let her husband grieve as well. "There is a grieving process for every member of the family, even children, especially if they're old enough to recognize what's going on," Kathy says. She believes that her marriage is stronger today because she and her husband took time to acknowledge that her illness had changed their lives. I like Linda Welsh's suggestion that we make a list of everything we believe we have lost, and express our grief for each one.[10] When we do this as a couple, however, we have to be careful not to blame each other. That's likely to inflame our passions and pull us apart rather than bring us together.

Talking to Each Other.   As a couple, we need to find a way of talking about the impact that chronic illness has on our lives in such a way that each partner feels respected and cared for. This is more difficult than it sounds. For example, when I voice fears about my future earning potential, my husband thinks I'm asking him to work harder. When he paints a rosy picture of our lives together, I think he expects me suddenly to be well. My husband and I have had to learn to hear what the other has to say without imposing our own interpretation on it.

Sometimes it's difficult to talk about our illness in ways that our partner will understand. "With chronic fatigue syndrome, I'm always tired, so telling Gary I'm tired on any particular day can lose some of its meaning," Sally says. She and her husband developed a ten-point rating scale that gives them a shorthand way of describing how she feels. On their scale, one means being bedridden and ten represents a total absence of symptoms. Most days, Sally is a three or four, with five being a good day for her. In addition to helping her communicate more clearly with her husband, the scale also allows Sally to learn to pace herself. "If I'm having a three day, I can't expect to do certain things."

Dulce has developed ways to advise her husband that cognitive troubles are making it difficult for her to understand him. "I've learned to say, 'You must stop. My brain will not absorb that right now,'" Dulce says. Like Dulce, I find that I can't process certain information, particularly directions to a place I've never been, when I am not feeling well. My husband finds this especially puzzling. He has a hard time understanding that sometimes I truly cannot grasp what he is saying. I remember telling him one evening when we were dating that his ability to go on talking was outstripping my ability to continue listening. Forgetting that I was in my own home, I told him, "I have to go now." I knew he truly cared for me when he gave me a bemused smile and said, "I think that's my cue to leave."

Living with someone who is uncommunicative can strain my husband's patience, however. By the time he gets home from delivering newspapers on Sunday morning, he has a wealth of information to share with me. But I am at my foggiest in the morning, and it never fails to disappoint him that some days the best I can do is smile at him over the comics.

Realizing that Our Lives Have Changed.   Pinpointing Sally's health on a scale helps both her and Gary to understand their situation better. So too does Gary's belief that, in life, each of us bears a fifty-pound weight that symbolizes all of our responsibilities. When one partner has a chronic illness, he maintains, each carries an additional twenty-five pounds, representing the fact that they both work a little bit harder. "There is a tendency to look at the amount of objective work that each partner is doing," Gary told me. "For example, today I got up at 5:30 A.M., worked nine hours, and drove home. This evening, I'll wash the dishes and fold some laundry. Sally ran some errands and washed clothes, which objectively is less work than I did. But because of her illness, the same amount of effort on Sally's part yields less objective work. I think it's fair to say, however, that each of us is working equally hard to make our relationship succeed."

Sally finds it remarkable that Gary can look at their situation this way, rather than feeling that he alone carries the extra burden. She also realizes that his acceptance, like hers, is for today and not forever. Gary says he is happier now that he is not comparing himself to others, or to what his life might have been, a message he tries to get across to the members of his on-line caregivers group. "You can achieve a greater sense of peace if you focus on what you have," Gary says. "This is a constant fight, but it's a really big step you need to take."

Seeking Professional Help.   Many of the individuals I interviewed acknowledged that at one point or another they sought professional counseling to help strengthen their relationships. For some, the impetus was a personal or family crisis but invariably the impact of chronic illness was one of the topics they addressed. My husband and I have done much of the hard work of making our marriage succeed on our own, but we have also participated in a group sponsored by my HMO that teaches communication skills to couples. Though we were the only couple in our group for whom chronic illness was an issue, all of our related concerns, including money, were ones the other participants shared.

Having Fun Together.   Money woes, sexual problems, and getting the dishes done can take every bit of energy we have. Sometimes, we forget to have fun. Jeri and her husband have learned to be spontaneous. When her lupus symptoms are under control and she is having what she calls "overwhelming feelings of wellness," Jeri will call her husband at work and he'll take the day off to celebrate. Obviously, it isn't always possible for someone to drop everything to have fun with us but we need to make recreation a priority whenever and however we can. Chronic illness is hard work for us and for our partners, and we need to make time to play. "My husband can paint the porch floor another day," Jeri explains. "But I may not be able to pick apples again anytime soon." There was a time when her husband viewed her behavior as controlling, Jeri says, but now he understands the need to take full advantage of her good days.

Likewise, my husband enjoys taking weekend getaways whenever we can. Even though I like exploring new or favorite places with him, sometimes the effort of getting there is just too much for me. On a weekend when I wake up and say, "Let's take off," he no longer thinks twice. The long grass and dirty clothes will be waiting when we return.

When we can't do things with them, those of us who are ill may need to encourage our partners to get out on their own. "It must be awful to have rearranged your schedule and made plans to go canoeing and then have your spouse wake up ill that day," Jeri acknowledges. "We can suggest that our family go canoeing by themselves, but they don't want to go by themselves, they want to go with us." Although they are disappointed, family members might better go alone than stay home and resent us for spoiling their fun. "You don't need to compound your spouse's suffering by increasing your own or denying yourself pleasure because your spouse can't enjoy it," Linda Welsh writes. "What really happens is that the pain is doubled, rather than shared, by mutual suffering and deprivation."[11] To stave off feelings of being left out, we can use this time to do something nice for ourselves. When my house is quiet, I like to pop a big bowl of popcorn that I don't have to share and watch an old movie. A bubble bath, a good book, or a long talk with a friend also can take the edge off feeling alone.

PARENTING WITH CHRONIC DISEASE

"Short on experience and long on dependence, a change in family dynamics is a relative revolution in the life of a child," Dr. Jeff Kane writes in *Be Sick Well*.[12] Parenting with a chronic illness can be overwhelming for moms and dads, too. Those of us who are ill feel inadequate because we can't play ball or walk through a fair or amusement park. Our partners may bear more of the physical work of child rearing, from changing diapers to teaching our sons and daughters how to ride a bike. Both parents and children have to make an extra effort to understand one another's concerns.

Explaining What's Wrong

The most important fact we need to know is that we can't fool our kids. If we do, Miryam Williamson reminds us, they may imagine the worst. "My biggest regret in raising my children is that I wasn't always there for them the way they needed me to be, and I couldn't tell them why," Miryam told me. Though she remembers being in pain from the age of five, and was quite ill when her children were young, Miryam didn't receive a diagnosis of fibromyalgia until she was fifty-seven years old and her three children were grown. "I wish I had been able to explain to them what was going on," she says. She wonders if they might have had fantasies about her dying. Because they had to help her, Miryam says, her children have grown up to be independent and competent adults. Still, it has only been in the last several years that she and her children have been able to clear up some misunderstandings. "My oldest daughter suffered more from it and, to some extent, still feels a little let down that we didn't have the family she wanted to have."

I know that one of the most concrete memories of childhood for my teenage son will be that his mother was tired all the time, and that makes me sad. Indeed, he has told me that he was both angry and afraid that I didn't have more energy. Perhaps it's a rationalization, but I like to think my lack of physical stamina helped in one regard: too tired some days to both clean house and play with my son, I would spend hours sitting on the floor with him building wooden towers and watching endless reruns of his favorite video.

Encouraging Questions

We need to keep our children informed and encourage them to ask questions, Linda Welsh says.[13] This comes naturally to Wendy Hay, who says she has never talked down to her boys, ages eight and four. She doesn't hide the fact that she injects medication to keep her multiple sclerosis symptoms at bay, and she answers their concerns in age-appropriate ways. "We explained to my older son that when Mommy's brain sends a message to her hand or her leg, sometimes it gets lost," Wendy says. "Of course, there's a new question every day, and we always try to answer it the best we can." Her younger son is not quite old enough to understand why his mom can't play outside some days but, overall, Wendy says that both her boys are a big help. "They fold laundry, 'wash' dishes, offer to scratch my back, ask me how I'm feeling and, most importantly, they act like any eight- and four-year-old boys."

Kelly sometimes worries that her children are growing up too fast. "My son tells people that Mommy has hurting arms and hurting legs," Kelly says. "That's how he describes my illness." At age six, he's the sensitive one, sitting on her lap and stroking her hair if she looks tired or sad. Kelly's ten-year-old daughter takes care of Mom, reminding her to wear sunscreen and a hat to avoid a lupus flare. "Sometimes I go to bed and cry because she is acting older than she needs to," Kelly says. Still, she thinks her children are more sensitive to others as a result of understanding her needs.

Empowering Our Children to Be Part of the Solution

Sharing information about our disease may help our children feel included when difficult decisions need to be made. One night, when her thirteen-year-old daughter was in sixth grade, Kathy Hammitt was up late reading medical articles on lymphoma. For the second time in little more than a decade, her rheumatologist suspected she had developed cancer of the lymph system, a rare complication of Sjogren's syndrome. "My daughter stayed up with me and helped me pore over those articles," Kathy says. "I don't look at that as something that was horribly traumatic for her because I was making her part of the solution. She was able in the same way I was to take control of the situation." Kathy acknowledges this might not be the best way for everyone to handle a similar situation but suggests it is an option we have. Before we share specific details about our illness with our children, we need to gauge their maturity level and their ability to handle potentially upsetting information.

Learning Not to Be Overprotective

More than anything else, our children need to know that their primary job is to be kids. But trying too hard to protect them from our situation doesn't serve anyone well. Linda Welsh says she tried to shield her son and daughter from the harsh realities of their father's battle with kidney disease. "My need to protect my children often kept me from asking for their help," she writes. "In doing so, I was being disrespectful to their capabilities and denying them a chance to feel useful."[14]

Likewise, I tried to hide my growing health problems from my son. I wanted him to have the same life that all his suburban friends had, and I was determined not to let ill health or the fact that I was a single parent stand in my way. I served as a Cub Scout den mother and sat in the wind and the rain at Little League baseball games. I also did the bulk of the cooking and cleaning, even when my son became old enough to help. When pain and fatigue began to limit my endurance, I asked my son to take more responsibility for himself so that I could take care of me. At first, I thought that needing his help meant I was failing as a parent. But as I saw my son grow into his new role, I realized that my overprotectiveness had stifled both his growth and my own recovery. Today, at age fifteen, my son's increasing sense of independence is a delight to both of us.

Helping Our Children Express Emotions

Initially, my son was angry that I expected more from him, and he was angry that I was ill. He also was afraid about what would happen to me, and, by extension, to himself. For a time when he was younger, he refused to visit his father on alternate weekends because he thought he needed to be home to take care of me. When I assured him that I would be fine on my own, he felt free to go on being a kid.

Just as we and our partners experience intense and sometimes conflicting emotions, so too do our children. But depending on their age, and on the family's style of coping, they may have little experience recognizing or expressing their feelings. If we keep a stiff upper lip, our children will too, Linda Welsh believes. "It is imperative, even when they are too young or too afraid, that children verbalize their feelings, and that you help them articulate feelings such as resentment, abandonment, anger, jealousy, a need for attention, fear of hurting a parent, or guilt," she says.[15] Sometimes younger children won't be able to talk about their emotions, but they can be encouraged to draw or to act out some of their bad feelings.

Without planning to, my son and I developed what I like to call "balloon therapy." Cleaning up after a party, we decided to pop the leftover balloons. Before we did, we took a felt-tip marker and labeled them with things we didn't like. My son, who was eight years old at the time, asked me how to spell "arthritis" to write it on one of his balloons. I wrote "being tired" on one of mine. As we exploded the balloons, we symbolically banished these unwanted visitors from our lives.

We know our kids best, and if we notice significant changes in their behavior, such as not caring about their homework or acting out at home or at school, we may need to seek professional help. Often, however, when we give our children the time and the emotional freedom they need to come to terms with our illness, we find they can be creative and capable in ways we never imagined.

Caring for Children Who Are Sick

Few things are more heartbreaking to a parent than to have a sick child. Caring for a chronically ill child when we are sick ourselves intensifies our emotions and our physical pain. Pam's fourteen-year-old daughter has chronic fatigue syndrome and, like her mother, fibromyalgia. When their local school district could no longer accommodate her daughter's frequent absences, Pam sent her to live with relatives in another town. There, the school system lets her work at home at her own pace. Pam says that not living with her only child is "excruciating," especially when her own health problems conspire to keep them apart. "I don't travel well, I need regular sleep, and I never know when my irritable bowel will act up, so I can't go to see my daughter during the week," Pam told me. Mother and child keep in touch by E-mail and by phone. "Having less pressure about school has relieved some of her symptoms," Pam says, "and I'm not ignoring my own needs to take care of her."

When Having Children Is Not an Option

Some of us become ill before we become parents. Though chronic illness need not be a barrier to pregnancy and to parenting, we may find we just don't have the energy. "I grew up assuming that I would have children," Sally told me. "I saved some of my toys and books, and I kept my favorite childhood jewelry, thinking that my daughter would wear it some day." But with chronic fatigue syndrome, Sally feels ill prepared to care for a child when, some days, she has all she can do to take care of herself. She says, "I can't even consider being a mother at this point." The loss of the family that might have been is yet another dream we may have to set aside.

Confronting Pregnancy Risks

Sometimes we decide that the importance of having a child outweighs the potential risks involved. Kathy Hammitt has a healthy son who was born after her diagnosis of Sjogren's syndrome, though she is well aware of the possible complications she and her son might have faced. Testifying in 1991 before an NIH task force on the need for research in women's health, Kathy noted, "Women with Sjogren's face an increased risk of miscarriage, a 30 percent chance of flare-up with the major hormonal changes of pregnancy, and the threat of fetal heart block."[16] According to the Sjogren's Syndrome Foundation, fetal heart block occurs when autoantibodies in the mother's blood attack the fetus's developing heart tissue, resulting in an abnormal heartbeat.[17] As a result, Kathy told the NIH group, some babies die in utero or in the first year of life, while others survive with or without a pacemaker. To help other women make an informed choice about whether or not to become pregnant, and to be certain they get appropriate prenatal care, Kathy served for many years as the Sjogren's Syndrome Foundation's contact person for prospective mothers.

Women who have fibromyalgia may experience a remission of their symptoms during pregnancy, followed by a flare-up after birth, Miryam Williamson writes.[18] The role of female hormones as both a protective factor and a causative agent in certain chronic diseases is only now beginning to be investigated.

Remembering to Have Fun

Just as we must remember to have fun with our spouses, so too in spite of or perhaps because of our illnesses we must remember to have fun with our children. Children bring joy into our lives even when chronic illness forces us to work extra hard to be the kind of parents we want to be. I'm an avid movie fan, and this is something my son and I can enjoy together even when I'm not feeling well, thanks to video rentals. We can involve our children in being creative about ways to spend time together. When our children are young, we can take turns reading to each other, find pictures in the clouds, or have an impromptu picnic in the backyard or even in the living room. The latter was a big hit with my son on a rainy day. As they get older, our sons and daughters may enjoy reading us a poem they wrote for English class, helping us plan the menu for a family meal, or flipping through photo albums of their younger years. Despite my fears about being an inadequate parent, I thank God every day for my son, who never fails to make me laugh just when I need to the most.

OUR PARENTS' CHILDREN

Though most of us are grown and on our own when we become sick, we still crave our parents' love and approval. A few of us have experienced the kind of unconditional love that gives us a wonderful model of caring for ourselves and for our own children. But many of us received negative messages as a child, and this affects the way we feel about ourselves and our disease.

Modeling Strength

Lois Arias considers her mother to be a pillar of strength. From the time Lois was a child, Lois says, her mother taught her not to give in to adversity or wallow in misery. When Lois's first husband died and later, when she developed interstitial cystitis, Lois followed her mother's example. "Sometimes you have to collapse, otherwise you're not owning up to your feelings," Lois told me. "But after you feel sorry for yourself, you've got to pick yourself up and say, 'Okay, I had a good pity-party, and it's time to get on with life.' " She's passed this attitude on to her son. At the tender age of four and a half, he's shown an active interest in his mom's on-line support community, and he recently acquired some pen pals of his own, including a six-year-old girl who has interstitial cystitis. Lois says, "He knows that when things go wrong, feeling bad doesn't make you better."

Mixed Messages

I received mixed messages about being sick when I was young. Because my mother was often ill, leaving me to help care for my younger brother, I came to regard sickness as a nuisance that more often than not interfered with my plans. But I also saw that being sick confers special benefits on the person who is ill, such as being able to stay in bed and have things done for you. To this day, I vacillate between wanting to have someone take care of me when I'm not feeling well and being annoyed with myself that illness is slowing me down. Neither attitude is conducive to healthy self-care.

Counteracting Negative Messages

Lois's mother gave her a clear and positive message about handling life's ups and downs, and she and her mother are very close. But those of us who received negative feedback from our parents may find it hard to repair strained relationships, especially if we were admonished for behaviors that may have been early signs of our disease. "When I was little, my mother used to say, 'Dulce is the only person I've ever seen who can be standing perfectly still and fall down,'" Dulce told me. In addition to balance problems associated with fibromyalgia, Dulce experienced cognitive difficulties, often having trouble finding the right word. Sometimes she made up words to substitute for ones that eluded her or turned her malapropisms into a joke. In doing so, she learned to laugh at herself, something that people admire her for today.

Like Dulce, I also was teased for being uncoordinated when I was growing up, as well as for needing to use a bathroom frequently. Clearly, my family didn't know that I would become ill later in life or that some of my idiosyncracies might actually be symptoms of disease. Still, I remain fairly sensitive to certain comments. On a good day, I can laugh with those who wonder how small my bladder must be. But if I'm really not feeling well, I let them know this topic is off-limits.

Sally has taken a more direct approach to explaining chronic fatigue syndrome to her family. Often chided when she was growing up for being so tired, she has decided to be clear with them about the reality of her disease. "I no longer defend my disease to my family any more than I would if they tried to tell me I'm not female," Sally says. "I know that I'm a woman. I know the sky is blue. I know that I have chronic fatigue syndrome."

This behavior allows Sally to take care of herself and it also helps her family to accept her needs better, according to her husband, Gary. The last time the couple visited Sally's parents, she was very clear about the fact that she would have to take a daily nap and be in bed early. When she stated her needs this way, her family respected them. "I found to my surprise that our families were in large part taking their cues from us, because they don't deal with chronic illness every day," Gary told me. "They look to us to see how to act."

Pam says her mother was better able to understand her struggles with fibromyalgia when she developed it herself. "The big breakthrough was the day my mom phoned and told me she had been diagnosed with fibromyalgia," Pam says. The fact that Pam, Pam's daughter, and Pam's mother all share similar symptoms has opened up lines of communication. "I know it could have done the reverse," Pam says, "but instead, we share coping mechanisms." None of us would wish our illnesses on anyone, least of all our parents or our children, but Pam's story illustrates that sometimes our families may not understand what we are saying because they have no appropriate frame of reference. When we talk about brain fog or dry eyes or muscles that won't cooperate, we truly are speaking a foreign language.

Coping with Rejection

Where many of our families do not fully understand or accept our disease, some totally reject the notion that we are ill. Angela was adopted as an infant by her biological aunt. Her adoptive mother was completely unable to accept the fact that Angela had multiple sclerosis. "She was unwilling to acknowledge that one of her children was less than perfect," Angela told me. "In the last years of her life, she completely rejected me. She did not want to be seen in public with her crippled daughter, and she would not acknowledge that I needed to use a wheelchair. She assumed that I was doing it as a sympathy ploy." Her mother's reaction to her disease was not the only troubled spot in Angela's relationship with her but it was the problem that erected a permanent barrier between them. Angela was resigned to her mother's attitude but sad that it kept them apart, especially when her mother died.

Sometimes we sense rejection in less obvious ways. Family members may not accept our need to turn down an invitation, or they may change the subject when we want to talk about our disease. Clinical social worker Cindy Perlin frequently sees people who are sick whose families disbelieve them or show a lack of concern. "This behavior retraumatizes those individuals whose needs may have been neglected when they were children," Perlin says. "Their families' reaction reopens old wounds, which causes more stress, grief, and anger, and may interfere with the patients' healing."

I like Miryam Williamson's suggestion that we write or tape-record a message to our families, and then throw the letter away or erase the tape.[19] Having done that, she says, we can talk about our disease without rancor. Some of us discuss family issues with a professional therapist, learning ways to accept ourselves in the face of outward criticism or rejection. Like Sally, we may find that when we acknowledge our own needs, our families will too, even if they don't fully understand them.

A FRIEND FOR ALL SEASONS

Many of us turn instinctively to our friends when we need support. We share heartaches and joys with our longtime friends, and we talk about the rituals of everyday life with friends we know from work, church, and school activities. Some of these friends will stick with us through our illness, but others will fall away.

Educating Our Friends

"You've got to be willing to educate your friends about your disease," Angela says. "They're not going to know anymore about it than you do, and they're not in your body. You can't expect that people will understand that because you're sick, you can't do certain things." We need to be explicit about what our disease will mean for our relationships, such as our inability to make plans too far in advance or our need to cancel activities on a moment's notice. Also, we have to be willing to let some of our friends go.

"They're not bad people," Angela says. "They just can't deal with our illness." We may lose friends because they are afraid our disease is contagious, because we can no longer share a sport or hobby with them, or because we don't seem to be as much fun as we used to be. Sometimes our friends just don't know how to act around us when we are ill. "When I tell people I have multiple sclerosis, they say, 'Oh, I'm sorry,' and they want to get away as fast as they can because they don't know what to say," Wendy Hay told me. Others treat her with kid gloves. Wendy says these responses are similar to the ones she got when she told friends that her mother had died unexpectedly. Death is an appropriate metaphor for chronic illness. When we become sick, the person our friends knew has died, and they may not know how to relate to the one who takes his or her place.

Sometimes our circle of friends becomes smaller when we are ill because we just don't have the energy to maintain multiple relationships. I find that I'm able to keep up with those friends who are equally likely to stay in touch with me. When I feel that I'm doing most of the work to maintain a friendship, I quietly and gently let it go.

Adjusting Our Expectations

Explaining our illness to our friends who are not sick doesn't necessarily mean sharing all the intimate details. For example, Linda Webb notes, "Talking about your bowels is not socially acceptable." We may need to readjust our expectations of the kinds of support that our friends reasonably can be expected to provide.

Mireille felt betrayed because she thought her "true" friends would understand her struggles with fibromyalgia, but a number of them drifted away when she was no longer able to join them in social activities. "I've now given up this need to have everyone understand how I feel," Mireille says. "I think my need to explain myself must have been a little difficult to take." Mireille values those friends who don't mind going to the movies on a moment's notice or going by themselves if she can't make it. She also has adjusted her expectations of herself. "I don't worry that people will see me as less of a person if I can't do something with them. I might say something simple like, 'I turn into a pumpkin after 6 P.M.' People usually laugh, and some admit that they do too." Being honest with our friends allows them to be honest with us.

Treasuring Best Friends

Many of us have learned to say we're "fine" when we know that a longer explanation would not be appropriate or accepted. Because of this, we treasure those friends to whom we can pour out our heart. Lexiann Grant-Snider has such a friend in Denise Tucker, who lived across the street from her when both girls were in second grade. Lexiann is an only child, and Denise has three brothers. The two have been as close as sisters for the past thirty-three years, even when Lexiann lived more than two hours away. Now, the two friends live ten minutes apart, and they talk for at least an hour every day. "We never run out of things to talk about," Denise told me.

Lexiann is grateful for Denise's unconditional support, but she is aware of the limitations of the friendship nonetheless. "Even Denise doesn't understand what I go through," Lexiann says, "though she never criticizes or complains, and she takes the friendship for exactly what it is." Denise acknowledges that she can't really know what Lexiann experiences. "I trust what she tells me because she has no reason to lie to me, but I don't really know how she feels," she says. Denise admits she gets frustrated when Lexiann cancels plans at the last minute, even though she knows that possibility always exists. Also, she wishes Lexiann would push herself harder. "Sometimes I think she rests too much and that makes her more tired," Denise says.

Though the two friends don't always see eye to eye, their friendship has lasted as long as it has because both provide what the other needs within their limitations. Denise says she doesn't always know what to say about Lexiann's health problems, but she knows she can listen and be her friend. In turn, Denise knows she can count on Lexiann to listen to her troubles as well. When the two friends get together, Denise says, "We laugh to keep from crying."

Like Lexiann, I am privileged to have a long-term friendship that has spanned nearly thirty years. My best friend always accepts what I tell her about my health problems, even when it doesn't seem to make sense to her. When she recently became ill, she was able to empathize truly with some of what I've felt, and I could offer her the support of someone who has been there. But our respective health problems are only a small part of the fabric of our friendship, and that helps give me the perspective that I am much more than my disease. I value the time we talk about our children, the books we are reading, and our shared past as much if not more than any discussion we have about chronic illness.

To Tell or Not to Tell

With older friends, it can be hard to hide a change in our health or unnecessary to do so. But with newer friends, we sometimes struggle with the question of when to say we have a chronic illness and how much detail to reveal. "On the one hand, you feel like you're withholding information if you don't tell people you have a chronic illness, but on the other hand, there's a tendency to want to hold back because you don't want that to be the focus of your relationship," Kathy Hammitt says. "You want to be treated first for you, and not for the person with a chronic disease."

Like Lexiann, Kathy wants to know what is going on in her friends' lives as well. She feels sad when friends won't share their troubles because they feel that hers are worse. For this reason, she often hesitates to tell people that she has Sjogren's syndrome. Also, Kathy says, she's glad she doesn't look sick. Though people might take her symptoms more seriously, she says, "Looking sick really would set me apart, and then I couldn't sometimes pretend that I'm well."

Each time I told someone that I was writing a book about chronic illness and they wanted to know why I was interested in the topic, I held my breath. When I admit that I have chronic health problems, I feel as if I am walking out on a limb that may break without warning. Also, I notice that I try to sound as healthy as I can when I say that I'm sick, even if I'm having a terrible day! Thus far, I've been pleasantly surprised that no one seems to treat me any differently. Of course, this is a double-edged sword. Although most days I want to be treated like anyone else, there are times when I think it would be nice to have special privileges because I'm the one who is sick.

Handling Unsolicited Advice

At the opposite end of the spectrum from the friends who fall away are those who want to tell us how to manage our illnesses. Our friends want to do something to help us, and some believe that the least they can offer is free advice. Mireille calls these friends "fixer uppers," and she tries to avoid them whenever she can. "If you don't follow up on their well-meaning suggestions, or worse, don't get better following their advice, they feel they have failed you or you have failed them, which is not a good basis for a friendship." Most of us have been the recipient of unso-licited medical advice. Learning how to handle it gracefully is an impor-tant step in our own recovery.

"Accept with sincere gratitude whatever kind of help friends offer, even though you may believe it to be useless or even harmful," Dr. Jeff Kane advises.[20] We may find this hard to do until we are certain in our own minds that we are following the course of treatment that is best for us. Often, we may try to justify our actions to our friends when really we are trying to convince ourselves. Over time, we learn that we can reject others' ideas in a polite and lighthearted way. When my favorite aunt told me that my arthritis would improve if I stopped eating tomatoes and potatoes, I told her, half jokingly, that I would rather have arthritis. We laughed together, and our conversation moved easily to another topic.

Angela's reaction to unsolicited advice depends on the source. Some-times friends will suggest that she sleeps too much, or that by using the wheelchair she is further weakening her muscles. To those friends she thinks will understand, she explains why she takes a nap every afternoon. "For the most part," Angela says, "I just laugh it off and say that some of us are lazier than others." The more confident we feel about ourselves and our treatment plan, the more we can accept our friends' ideas about our health care with equanimity. We may even discover some good ideas in what they have to offer, and we can at least be grateful that they care enough to want to help.

Asking for What We Need

Our friends are not mind readers, psychologist Linda Welsh reminds us, and when we fail to ask for what we need, we deprive them of the op-portunity to help us.[21] Most of us consider ourselves to be independent people, and we have a hard time asking for what we need. Sometimes, in fact, Eileen finds it easier to be alone. "Being alone causes tremendous isolation, but it also is a relief because I'm not responsible for somebody else's needs," she says. She has a strong support system but without one person she can always count on, getting help is hit or miss. "I have to decide who I want to know that I'm scared," she says.

I'm more than guilty of holding onto the attitude that "I can do this myself," and it's been quite humbling to realize this isn't always true. I've had to learn to ask for help in small ways first. When I need to vent my frustration, I sometimes ask a friend to listen without offering a solution. I might even tell her what I need to hear. Indeed, I've been known to start a conversation by saying, "I'm going to describe my latest problem with (fill in the blank), and I want you to say, 'What a shame you have to go through this.' " The first few times I tried this, some of my friends felt they were being insincere by parroting my words. But they have come to appreciate that I don't expect them to know what I need, while I have the satisfaction of knowing they can offer the support I want.

Of course, we can try this with more concrete assistance as well. We might ask a friend to pick up clothes at the dry cleaners, take our child to the library, or stop for a cup of coffee when we're too tired to venture out. The worst they can say is no, and we may be pleasantly surprised at their willingness to lend a hand.

SETTING LIMITS

To preserve our energy and our relationships, we have to learn to set limits. First, this requires that we accept the fact that we do indeed have certain limitations we must respect. This is a constant battle for many of us. We can be very stubborn and insist on doing what we want when we want to, no matter the consequences to our health. At times I have been told by those who love me that I am exaggerating my pain when in reality I usually am exaggerating my health. Doing so helps no one, least of all me.

Learning to Say No

"The first thing I did when I found out I had multiple sclerosis was learn to say no," Wendy Hay told me. "Before that, I would promise to do something and then struggle trying to get it done." She admits that at first, it was hard to say no and not feel guilty. But she knew she needed to re-duce the stress in her life. When Wendy can't do something that someone asks of her, she lets them down gently. "I've learned to say, 'I'll *be* there for you, but I can't *do* that for you.' "

Like Wendy, we often find that saying no doesn't always feel good. We want to make our family and friends happy, but not at the expense of our health. Using humor can ease their disappointment. Mireille has de-veloped a clever way to let others know that she is not available for a visit. She has hung a sign on her townhouse door that reads as follows:

> BEFORE YOU KNOCK
> Please go to the lobby and dial my extension. If there's no answer, the phone is off because I need to rest.
> Lights on, or TV or radio sounds, are no indication I'm awake or up.
> Interrupting my required naps once too often can affect my sunny dis-position. ☺
> Thank you in advance.

Her request has been well received. "My family and friends have fun with this, teasing me when they visit, but it has worked beautifully so far," Mireille says. "Everyone has followed the instructions, even the census taker, who told me he wouldn't want to disturb my sunny disposition!"

Taking Care of Ourselves

Many of us discover it's not only our own desire to help others or to do things for ourselves that gets in the way of setting appropriate limits. We may find that our family thinks it's fine for us to take care of ourselves as long as their needs have been met. Women in particular have a hard time putting themselves first. In her social work practice, Cindy Perlin ad-vises women with chronic illness that taking care of themselves is practi-cal rather than selfish.

"Whether you have cancer or you have chronic headaches, you have to think about the impact on your family if you get sicker," Perlin tells clients. "It's better not to wait until you're too sick to do anything, but to learn to say to your family, 'I need to do this so I can be healthy and be there for you the rest of the time.' " Perlin says this is a process, not a one-time event. "You have to get people used to the idea that you are going to be taking care of yourself," she points out. Further, your family can't nec-essarily be expected to like the idea. "Any change you make in family dy-namics will upset the balance," Perlin says. "Family members will resist the change, and you'll keep getting pulled in because of habit or guilt." We have to learn to stand our ground if we want to be taken seriously.

Stopping Before It's Too Late

If our family and friends have a hard time understanding our limits, it may be because we do too. When we feel well, we want to do all the work or have all the fun we've been putting off for a better day. We may not realize until a day or two later that we overextended ourselves.

Gary used to think that people with chronic fatigue syndrome, like his wife, Sally, overexerted themselves because they didn't have an accurate perception of their resources at any given time. After talking with other spouses and caregivers, he now believes that social pressure is a bigger part of the problem. "No one wants to be sick or have to admit to themselves that they can't meet others' expectations," Gary says. Also, we want to be able to have fun like anybody else. Sometimes it just doesn't seem fair that many of the things I truly enjoy, such as weekend getaways with my husband, take so much out of me. Reluctantly, I've had to learn to parcel out my energy carefully. I can decide to spend my energy all at once, but I must build in time to recoup it later.

LOVING OURSELVES, LOVING OTHERS

Chronic illness throws a monkey wrench into our relationships. We may seem as foreign to the people who love us as if we had begun speaking a different language. Our family and friends still want us to be the mom who works, the dad who plays baseball in the backyard, and the friend who meets them for lunch. In turn, we want to be treated as the same loving spouse, parent, and friend we always have been. A large part of the responsibility for making these relationships work falls to us. We have to educate our family and friends about our disease, allow them to express their emotions openly, and clearly state our limits and our needs. Also, we have to expect these changes to be unsettling.

Ultimately, as we strike a delicate balance between our own needs and the demands of our most important relationships, we grow in self-awareness, creativity, and acceptance. We can't be sick successfully without learning to love ourselves, and when we accept our own limitations, we're much more likely to let those around us be less than perfect too.

CHANGING THE WAY
WE LOOK AT WORK

Work is love made visible.
KAHLIL GIBRAN

Writing is more than what I do to make a living. Being a writer is *who I am*. Tying my sense of identity to what I do is at the heart of my struggles with chronic illness and work. Who will I be if I am no longer able to write?

Most of us need to work. We have to pay our bills, put our children through school, and plan for our old age. If we're not covered on someone else's health insurance plan, we need the benefits our jobs may provide. But the need for money is only part of the picture. Work helps define our place in the world. When pain, fatigue, or cognitive problems make it difficult for us to continue at our former pace, we face some difficult and painful choices. The way we approach these choices is a reflection of how well we accept ourselves and our disease.

In this chapter, we'll examine how difficult it can be to remain on the job and try to cover up our growing disabilities. We'll also explore the connection between work and self-esteem and discuss our right to special accommodations, such as a more comfortable chair or a reduced workload, that allow us to remain productive as long as we can. The phrase "reasonable accommodations" has a very specific meaning according to the Americans with Disabilities Act (ADA), and we'll discuss both our rights and our responsibilities under the ADA. We'll also highlight the long and often arduous process of applying for Social Security Disability Insurance (SSDI). Finally, we'll talk about the benefits and pitfalls of self-employment, which offers flexibility but also comes with long hours, unpredictable income, and a lack of paid sick leave or medical insurance.

Most importantly, we'll discover that we can define ourselves by *who we are* rather than by *what we do*. Striking a balance between our career aspirations and the need to protect our health is a key ingredient in our recovery.

BEING SICK ON THE JOB

The majority of us work for a living. Of 170 women eligible to participate in the fibromyalgia treatment program at OHSU, 60 percent were working outside the home, according to professor of nursing Carol S. Burckhardt. This is the national norm for women ages thirty to sixty, Burckhardt says. At the end of the six-month program, many of the 104 participants were working more rather than fewer hours, though some had changed jobs to find less stressful work.[1]

I have yet to meet a person with a chronic disease who isn't ambitious and hard driving. The people I interviewed are or have been Wall Street brokers, presidential campaign managers, news producers, graphic designers, newspaper reporters, psychotherapists, disability advocates, and business owners. Based on what we know about the effects of stress on the human immune system, we might suppose that our high-pressure jobs contribute to or exacerbate our illnesses. Indeed, this may be the case. But the reverse is also true. The fact that we have a disease that limits our capabilities makes us work especially hard. We might need more time to complete a project, but we always get it done. To meet others' expectations, as well as our own, we come in early, skip lunch, and take work home. While we are still well enough to pass as healthy, many of us go to elaborate lengths to cover up our symptoms.

Passing as Healthy

Pretending to be well when we are not takes precious energy we may not have to spare. For many of us, the phrase "I gave at the office" means that we use all of our personal resources between 9 A.M. and 5 P.M., leaving little or nothing else for a personal or family life. Eileen recalls that on her worst days, she would drive by the pharmacy on her way home from work without stopping to pick up medication she needed. She skipped dinner and didn't answer the phone. Teaching fourth grade and dealing with the symptoms of interstitial cystitis took all the energy she had. She didn't have anything left to give away.

Mornings can be especially difficult for those of us who wake up fatigued and in pain, making it a struggle just to get to work. On a typical day, my joints are stiff and swollen when I first get out of bed. My eyes are too dry to focus well, and my mouth feels as if it's stuffed with cotton. Often, my thinking is clouded for the first few hours I'm awake. If this were a hangover, at least I'd have something fun to remember from the night before.

When I was working at my last full-time job, writing and designing newsletters, I would shower and dress, get my son off to school, and drive thirty-five minutes in rush-hour traffic. Many days, I arrived at the office exhausted and close to tears. I was frustrated at my lack of stamina and afraid of being "found out." When I mentioned this to Eileen, she told me about a very vivid, recurring dream she had in which the school superintendent came into her classroom and found her in bed in her nightgown. We wear ourselves out trying to appear "normal," and we worry that our bosses and colleagues can see right through us.

High Pressure and Little Flexibility

Taking care of ourselves at work may be an elusive goal. Sometimes the nature of the job just won't allow it. Before her son was born, Lois Arias was a videotape editor for a major television network. She had frequent bladder infections, but if she was working with an on-air assignment she couldn't leave to go to the bathroom. "I think that could have aggravated my symptoms," says Lois, who subsequently was diagnosed with interstitial cystitis. Eileen had to find a way to keep a room full of fourth graders busy while she made numerous trips to the rest room.

Sometimes, we find ourselves in a job that is too high pressured for our diminished energies. Kathy Hammitt thrived on the challenge of being a news producer for a television network affiliate. It was not unusual for her to work weekends or stay up all night finishing a job. When her daughter was born and she began experiencing fever, weakness, and pain that later would be attributed to Sjogren's syndrome, Kathy realized she could no longer do her job well. "I couldn't work with both a child and a chronic illness," she told me. "It's hard enough with one of these." She wanted to focus her energy on getting well and taking care of her child. Kathy, who has a master's degree in journalism, and her husband, who is a lawyer, now run their own business publishing a newsletter and reference materials about the Freedom of Information Act.

Like Kathy, I have always tried to reserve enough energy to care for my son. I left a job I enjoyed as director of public relations for a private high school for girls in part because I didn't have enough stamina to be a good parent and to attend the evening and weekend functions that my position demanded. Frequently, when we have no choice but to tackle a difficult assignment, we call on all the resources we can muster, but we pay for it later. When Miryam Williamson managed a presidential primary campaign, she planned in advance to spend time in bed when it was over. She knows that, for her, running on adrenaline always brings on a fibromyalgia flare.

When We Can't Think Clearly

The cognitive dysfunction that accompanies many chronic illnesses, and that can be slightly embarrassing or even funny in social situations, can be a serious problem on the job. Those of us who experience cognitive difficulties as part of such illnesses as chronic fatigue syndrome, fibromyalgia, lupus, and Sjogren's syndrome may have trouble concentrating, understanding abstract concepts, or solving problems. It takes energy to overcome these deficits, and we worry that an especially noticeable lapse might cause our co-workers and bosses to wonder if we are up to the job. Eileen considers herself lucky to have had sympathetic students. She often would forget their names, but if she stared at them, they would clue her in.

Short-term memory problems associated with Lyme disease mean that Joan O'Brien-Singer, a substance abuse counselor for a nonprofit agency, can remember what clients told her three years ago but may not recall, without relying on her notes, what they discussed yesterday. Memory lapses, or what Joan calls "brain farts," have caused her to substitute descriptive phrases for clinical terms when discussing a client in a staff meeting. For instance, she has said, "when you are happy one minute and sad the next," when she can't recall the term *manic depression*. Mental confusion makes it hard for Joan to sense the relationship of one thing to another, so that collating even a small document becomes an arduous task on a bad day. "I can be sitting at the table crying because I don't know which page comes first," Joan says. "I can count, but somehow when I see the pages spread out before me, I can't put them together." We're notoriously hard on ourselves; after all, people who don't have a chronic disease may have these problems too. But what others attribute to having too much on their mind or advancing age, we take as further evidence of the fact that we are less than we used to be.

Sometimes, cognitive problems are less dramatic but no less frustrating. I make my living using words, and on days when I can't seem to string those words together into a coherent thought, I tend to panic. Panicking takes energy away from my work, so I have had to train myself to keep writing, knowing that I can edit my thoughts on a better day. I call this the vegetable soup method of writing—I throw everything in the pot one day, and I skim off the fat the next. When my thinking is especially fuzzy, I may have to take a short walk or a nap, which I am able to do since I've become self-employed. I also have learned to do those things that take less mental acuity, such as making phone calls or organizing files, when I can't write. In essence, my illness has taught me to work smarter, but I usually feel spent at the end of the working day. The running joke in my home is that my brain turns itself off at 5 P.M.

Straining the Sympathy of Bosses and Colleagues

Having a chronic illness doesn't give us a ready excuse on the job. In fact, with the bottom line in mind, our supervisors need us to produce as much if not more than we always have. Often we find that the people with whom we spend the bulk of our daytime hours are uninterested or even hostile about our disease. Our co-workers may disbelieve that we are ill, resent any special accommodations we receive, or even be frightened by the changes they see in us.

When the removal of dental fillings was touted as the cure for everything from chronic headaches to multiple sclerosis, one of my co-workers blithely advised me to have all of my fillings removed. I'm sure she meant well, but I also think she was tired of hearing me complain about symptoms that made me tired, cranky, and confused. When I cut my working hours from full-time to three-quarter time to accommodate my worsening health, I was vaguely aware that some of my office mates seemed jealous that I left at 3 P.M. every day. I would rather have felt better and worked until 5 P.M.

Of course, few situations are black and white. Though some of my colleagues seemed to resent my new hours, my supervisor and the head of the company were very supportive. They easily approved my change in hours, though I didn't seem to lose any of my responsibilities as a result! Cramming eight hours of work into six left me ready for a nap when I got home.

Pam was promoted to a supervisory position in the government agency for which she worked. But she missed so much time because of undiagnosed fibromyalgia that she frequently was subject to disciplinary action and eventually accepted the best of the options presented to her— she returned to her previous union job. Her manager had known Pam for eleven years and supported her desire to keep working as long as possible. "She knew that I wasn't faking it," Pam says, "because if I were, I was doing a real fine job of remembering to do the same things every day."

Some of Pam's colleagues were frightened by her deterioration while others were interested in knowing more about her condition. When her office was reorganized and Pam didn't feel well enough to find a new position, she allowed herself to be laid off.

Sally found that the academic world was not prepared to handle the needs of a student with chronic fatigue syndrome. She took ten years to complete her doctorate in clinical psychology and often was in trouble with the graduate curriculum committee. "They even put me on probation a number of times," Sally recalls. "They said they had their timetables and I just wasn't meeting them." When she served her residency, she had a difficult time finding a program that would accept her on a half-time basis, which was all that she could manage. Now that she has her degree, Sally worries that the work experience she needs before she can hang out her shingle will take years more to complete.

To Tell or Not to Tell

Because the reactions of supervisors and co-workers range from supportive to hostile, we may wonder whether to tell anyone at work that we are sick. Bob read a book about inflammatory bowel disorders that advised him not to talk about his disease at work lest his employer perceive him as someone who couldn't do the job. Despite what he read, Bob decided not to keep his diagnosis of Crohn's disease a secret from the editors at the daily newspaper where he is a reporter. This was helpful when he asked to reduce his workload during a flare-up of his illness. But Bob says he keeps the details of his disease to himself. "I don't talk about how good or bad I feel," he says.

Indeed, there are some compelling reasons to share the news about our health at work, Miryam Williamson writes. Like Bob, we will have an easier time seeking accommodations that allow us to continue working. Also, she notes, if there is a chance we will have to apply for disability, the fact that we have a chronic disease should appear on our work record.[2] Most importantly, we don't have to pretend to feel well when we don't.

The reasons against disclosure may be equally compelling. We may keep our health problems to ourselves for fear of losing out on choice assignments or being treated differently by our colleagues. On the one hand, I like it when clients who know that I am ill ask how I am feeling. But I'm uncomfortable when they inquire whether I'm capable of handling a job they have to offer. I want to be able to make that call. Part of the problem, of course, is that I may accept an assignment regardless of how I feel because I need the money or want to hold onto a good client. When I realize I'm in over my head, I rarely fail to meet my clients' needs but I certainly neglect my own.

I think Bob found the healthy middle ground in discussing his illness at work, and I wish I had discovered this earlier. At my last job, I mentioned my symptoms frequently, which may have made me sound as if I was whining, yet failed to let my employer know how my health was affecting my work. When I asked for a reduction in hours, my supervisor was surprised—she had no idea that I was feeling as poorly as I was. I could have improved the trust between us, and my own health, had I shared the bigger picture with her and kept the particulars to myself.

Inadequate Benefits

Even those of us who have fairly generous fringe benefits may find them inadequate to meet our need for time off. Ken Henderson used four more than his allotted twelve sick days, and even though he produced a doctor's note for every day he was out, his supervisor was preparing to fire him. Ken was too proud to let himself be fired, so he resigned, which made him ineligible to collect unemployment benefits. He understands the school district's need to have a reliable mechanic to keep its buses running but is upset that he lost his job because he has fibromyalgia. "If I had been doing something wrong that I could have corrected, that would have been different," he says. "I feel like I was punished for something I had no control over at all." Ken's new job, as a mechanic for the local subsidiary of a major oil company, doesn't offer paid sick leave. He's missed three days of work in his first six months on the job.

Now that I work for myself, nobody hassles me about taking time off, but I don't get paid for those days either. As a result, I rarely miss time from work. At my last job, I used most of my five sick days a year taking care of my son when he was home with a cold or an earache. When I did run over my allotted time, my employer let me take unpaid leave, but that may not be an option for some of us. Now that I'm self-employed, I also have to buy my own health insurance, a necessity I can't do without. I'm lucky to get a group rate through my local chamber of commerce, but that means I must pay $200 a year in dues to be a chamber member. And even at the group rate, medical and dental insurance cost me roughly $2,000 a year.

WORK AND SELF-ESTEEM

Loss of income and benefits is a significant reason to fear not working, especially if we are single or the family breadwinner. But many of us have a more profound dread about our growing inability to work. "To be occupied is essential," a former typist told Studs Terkel, author of *Working*. "I don't think man can maintain his balance or sanity in idleness. Human beings must work to create some coherence."[3]

Our reasons for valuing work may be very personal. Some of us have received messages as a child about the importance of hard work, or we may have inferred this meaning from our position and responsibilities in the family. When my mother was ill, I stepped into her role and cared for my younger brother. Further, my maternal grandmother often told me that if I didn't use the brains God had given me, I would lose the ability to do so. Being responsible and working hard became an essential part of my identity, especially when I discovered that the accolades I won in school brought positive strokes at home. I know that I haven't yet been able to let go of this picture of myself, but I don't think I realized how troubled I was by the change in my working life until I read this excerpt from one of the interviews I taped. Here's what I told one of my fellow fibromyalgia sufferers:

> I look at women who get dressed in their suits, put on their heels, and pick up their briefcases, and I think, 'I'm supposed to be like them, I'm such an intelligent person.' I know the effort of doing so would

exhaust me and make me miserable. *But I want to be that person.* Some days I long for the energy and the desire to present myself to the world as the intelligent, ambitious, and capable woman I know myself to be. I feel like a Type A personality trapped in a Type B body.[4]

Wasting Our Talents

Lexiann Grant-Snider captures this sentiment in a well-chosen phrase. "I feel like I've wasted my God-given talents," she told me. Lexiann has worked for a Fortune 500 company, owned a graphic arts business, and been director of development and public relations for a nonprofit agency. "I have not been physically able to work outside the home since 1988," says Lexiann, who has Sjogren's syndrome and hepatitis. Today, she has turned her love of dogs into a part-time business by selling articles freelance to national magazines for canine enthusiasts. Still, she says, "I could have been and done anything I wanted to before I got sick."

Societal as well as personal expectations come into play. Author Cheri Register, who has chronicled her battles with a rare congenital liver disease, writes, "In this culture, we measure our worth as human beings by the rewards we earn and the utility of the work we contribute to the common life. People who make no such contribution or whose work goes unpaid are hard put even to say who they are."[5]

"Who Will I Be?"

When we lose our health, we struggle to gain a new identity. While we are still working, we at least have the title of teacher or writer or businesswoman to fall back on. Losing that makes us feel like the last piece of our safety net has fallen away. Eileen was a fourth-grade teacher, in the same school, for twenty-eight years. When she and I met, she was struggling with her decision to retire. She told me, "When I stay home, I feel good. When I feel good, I think I can work. It's hard for me to pace myself." Her friends worried about what she would do with her time. "People ask me who I will be when I am no longer teaching," Eileen says. "I tell them I will be a retired teacher with other interests." Eileen decided to take early retirement, but she is hardly idle. She runs a local interstitial cystitis support group, and she has published historical plays for classroom use. When she's not working, Eileen says she has an acceptable quality of life.

What Is Life without Work?

Eileen struggled with her decision to retire, but Mireille felt she had no choice. When a back injury that kept her out of work for nearly two years flared again, she was forced to leave her position doing computer work for a small mental health agency, a job she loved. Previously, Mireille worked with developmentally disabled adults. In addition to her back problems, she has fibromyalgia.

"All of a sudden, I wondered, 'What is my life without work?'" Mireille told me. "Most of my social contacts were through work. I had friends but they worked also. I had no more purpose." Her doctor suggested she apply to the Canadian government for disability. When she went to apply, she discovered that "The forms are printed in both English and French, and the French word for disabled is *invalide*," Mireille says. "I didn't want to think of myself as disabled, first of all, and 'invalid' sounded like I was writing myself off." Her application was approved, and Mireille began a new phase of her life. Without the expectations of others to guide her, Mireille was left to figure out what she wanted to be and do. Today, she exercises, takes nature walks, and visits with her friends on the Internet. When others ask her what she does for a living, she replies lightheartedly, "As little as I can."

Redefining Ourselves

Like Mireille, Angela also worked in the field of developmental disabilities, and when multiple sclerosis forced her to leave work she was devastated. "I don't have children by choice," Angela says. "My identity was framed around being a working person. For about two years after I quit my job, I was deeply depressed, not so much because of the multiple sclerosis but because I was no longer contributing to my household or to life. I felt that meant I wasn't a good person."

Angela also was upset about the way she lost her job. She was employed by an agency whose philosophy is built on the notion that people with disabilities are entitled to the same rights as everyone else. "My boss knew that legally he couldn't fire me, so he was making it difficult for me to do my job," Angela says. "He made it quite clear that he would be happy if I left." After the job ended, not content to sit at home, she began to fill her life with volunteer activities. "I had to regain my own confidence that work should not define me," she says. Eventually, an agency for which Angela volunteered hired her as a consultant, which requires a lot of traveling. She throws her wheelchair in the back of her station wagon and visits offices around the state. "This agency has been incredible in their willingness to make whatever adaptations I need to do the job," Angela says. "They pay me to do a job I would do for free."

Afraid to Go Back

We may want to return to full-time work after a period of paid disability or a stint of self-employment. But when we've been out of the 9-to-5 routine for any reason, we wonder if we can ever go back. When I finally left full-time work three years ago, I immediately started to feel better. If I am having a bad day, I don't waste my energy pretending to feel well. I work harder now than I ever have, but I go at my own pace. When business is slow I think about going back to work for someone else, but the idea scares me. I don't know that I can maintain in a workplace setting the relative health I've found by being self-employed. I worry that I will end up in tears of frustration because I can't keep up and I can't keep covering up. Ultimately, striking a balance between the need to work and the need to be healthy is an ongoing process for me.

SEEKING ACCOMMODATIONS:
THE AMERICANS WITH DISABILITIES ACT (ADA)

Many of us who have a chronic illness are physically able to continue working though we may need some adjustments in the workplace environment to make that possible. Title I of the ADA, passed in 1990, ensures that we may seek reasonable accommodations to help us do our job, and the law requires that our employers respond to our requests. The ADA applies to all employers with fifteen or more employees.

Reasonable Accommodations

As defined by the ADA, a disability is a physical or mental impairment that substantially limits one or more of an individual's major life activities, including "caring for oneself, performing manual tasks, walking, seeing, hearing, speaking, breathing, learning, and working."[6] A reasonable accommodation is any modification or adjustment to the job application process or work environment that enables an individual with a disability to perform the essential functions of a position for which he or she is qualified.[7]

According to Francie Moeller, president of ADA Compliance Service in Guerneville, California, such accommodations may include buying a voice-activated computer for an employee who has trouble typing, restricting the amount of weight a person with a back injury has to lift, or modifying an employee's schedule to accommodate his or her need to work fewer hours. At my last job, to make it easier for me to design publications, the company purchased a trackball, a type of upside-down computer mouse. Holding my hand around a regular mouse aggravates my arthritis, but I can move the cursor with a trackball by using the tips of my fingers.

Accommodations can't infringe on other employees' rights, Moeller notes. For example, she explains, if you cannot tolerate perfume, you can't ask your co-workers not to wear it but you can wear a mask. Moeller, who has fibromyalgia and degenerative disk disease, has been trained by the Equal Employment Opportunity Commission (EEOC) and the U.S. Department of Justice to consult with and train lawyers, businesses, government agencies, and disability groups on the provisions of the ADA.

Undue Hardship

An employer cannot refuse to honor an individual's request for accommodation unless the company can prove that doing so would create an *undue hardship*. The ADA defines *undue hardship* as "any accommodation that would be unduly costly, extensive, substantial, or disruptive, or that would fundamentally alter the nature or operation of the business."[8] Depending on a company's size and resources, installing an elevator for a person who can't take the stairs might constitute an undue hardship, Moeller says. If the cost of an accommodation is prohibitive, the ADA requires an employer to allow the individual to provide it or to help the company pay for it.

Essential Functions

Further, an employer may not fire an otherwise qualified individual who requires a reasonable accommodation to perform the *essential functions* of a job. According to the legislation, a job function may be considered essential if the position exists to perform that function, if there are a limited number of employees among whom the performance of a job function can be shared, or if the individual is being hired for his or her expertise to perform a particular task.[9] The law prohibits an employer from imposing separate standards that would specifically exclude a person with a disability from meeting the essential functions of a position.

Legislating Attitudes

Most important to people with such illnesses as fibromyalgia and chronic fatigue syndrome, Francie Moeller says, "An employer cannot say they will not make a reasonable accommodation for you because they do not believe in your disease." Though a federal law protects us, however, we can't legislate people's attitudes. As *Houston Chronicle* reporter L. M. Sixel notes, "Employers tend to be more accommodating to people with well-known disabilities. People with less visible problems, such as mental illnesses, chronic fatigue syndrome, or neurological diseases, don't get as much employer support."[10]

Joan O'Brien-Singer is finding this to be the case with Lyme disease. A substance abuse counselor for a nonprofit agency, she is having trouble getting her boss to put things within her reach. Stiff joints make it difficult for her to bend down to retrieve office supplies or to store clients' urine samples for drug testing. "When I asked my boss to put the fax cover sheets in a place I could reach them, he said he wasn't going to rearrange the whole office for me." In addition, writing by hand is difficult for Joan, but she has little access to the computer and typewriter that are located on the secretary's desk. She is considering filing a complaint against her boss for ADA violations.

Filing a Complaint

Anyone can write an ADA complaint, which is filed with the EEOC, according to Francie Moeller. Indeed, she cautions us to be wary of someone who claims to be a "certified" ADA consultant, since there is no such certification process. It is good to find someone who knows the law, however, and Moeller says that many independent living centers—nonprofit groups that receive federal funds to aid people who are disabled—maintain a list of people who are knowledgeable about the ADA. In addition, you'll find some ADA resources, including toll-free telephone numbers and relevant Internet sites, listed in the resources section at the end of this book.

Individuals whose cases can't be resolved by the EEOC may file a lawsuit in federal court, but most complaints never get this far. Moeller says that of one thousand complaints she has written, only one made it all the way to court. Indeed, only 650 ADA lawsuits have been filed nation-wide in five years, according to the Department of Justice.[11] In part, Moeller says, this is because most accommodations are relatively inexpensive and easy to provide. Sears, one of the nation's largest retailers, reports that of 436 reasonable accommodations it provided between 1978 and 1992, 69 percent cost nothing, 28 percent cost less than $1,000, and only 3 percent cost more than $1,000.[12] We'll have better luck being successful with our requests for accommodations if we suggest solutions to our employer rather than just state problems, Moeller says. When I knew that I could no longer use a computer mouse, I researched alternatives to find an affordable trackball that would fit my workstation and relieve the pressure on my hand. I presented my recommendations to my supervisor, who authorized me to purchase the new equipment.

Seeking Employment

The ADA also protects individuals with disabilities who are seeking employment. According to the law, employers are forbidden from denying a position to a qualified individual who needs a reasonable accommodation to perform the essential functions of a job. Also, firms are prohibited from seeking medical information from an applicant prior to making an offer.[13] Once again, however, societal attitudes may not keep pace with legal rights. "At fifty years old, I found myself looking for work in a world where illness is not regarded as an asset on a job application," Ken Henderson says. He felt he had to be honest with prospective employers when they asked why he left his job with the school district. "I told them I resigned because of health problems, and they really didn't talk to me much past that." Living in a small town meant that Ken had limited choices for a new job, but it also may have been the reason he got his current position. His new employer heard that Ken had been forced to leave his last job and felt he had been treated unfairly. In fact, Ken still is able to handle the physical demands of vehicle maintenance when he is able to work.

Fighting Prejudice

Many of us find it hard to be thought of as less than a fully functioning human being. We're weighed down by personal and societal attitudes about work and prejudices about disability. "Like racism and sexism, there's 'handicapped-ism,'" Angela says. "We don't like people with handicaps because they look different. Those with invisible disabilities such as fibromyalgia or lupus get lumped into the same pool as soon as it's discovered that they have an illness. They'll find that attitudes start changing around them, too." When she started working in the field of disabilities, before she became disabled herself, Angela assumed that such attitudes would be easy to change. Today, she believes that prejudice is best addressed one person at a time. "The way people change their attitudes is to be around those of us with disabilities and discover that we have many of the same dreams and challenges in our lives as anyone else."

APPLYING FOR SOCIAL SECURITY DISABILITY INSURANCE (SSDI)

When working is no longer an option even with accommodations, our choices begin to narrow, and each of them has its drawbacks. We may want to take disability leave from our jobs to give ourselves time to heal physically and to explore new career possibilities. But aside from concerns about money, the first hurdle in seeking disability is accepting that we have a need, and a right, to do so. "Filing [for disability] is a tangible admission of the reality of the illness that calls a halt to any sort of denial," writes Janice Strubbe Wittenberg, a registered nurse who has chronic fatigue syndrome. "This can open the floodgates for you to grieve the loss of function, the loss of life-style, and the loss of self-definition."[14]

Depending on the type and the severity of our disease we may not feel we are entitled to collect disability payments, yet all of us who have worked have paid into the SSDI program to provide a safety net against potential loss of income. In addition, some of us have private disability insurance through our employers, though this likely will pay for a limited amount of time, such as one or two years and, if we receive partial disability from a private insurance program, we may waive our right to seek full disability in the future.[15]

Proving We Are Too Sick to Work

When we apply for reasonable accommodations under the ADA, we must prove to our supervisor, or to a prospective employer, that we are capable of doing a specific job with help. To receive government disability benefits, we must prove to the Social Security Administration (SSA) that we are incapable of doing any work for which we are suited, and that our disability is expected to last for at least a year or result in death.[16] "It is almost impossible to prove that you can't do anything," says Francie Moeller, who spent more than three years before she was able to get SSDI. She was turned down three times, saw seven doctors, and went through her savings in the process. Unfortunately, her experience is not unusual.

"The social security system does not easily or quickly rule favorably on a claim of disability," says Joshua W. Potter, a Pasadena, California, attorney who specializes in helping people with fibromyalgia obtain disability payments. "For patients with fibromyalgia and similar disease entities, whose very existence is often questioned, proof of disability is especially difficult."[17]

Proving that we are too sick to work may become a self-fulfilling prophecy, Janice Strubbe Wittenberg points out. "If you think of yourself as being disabled, you may become more disabled," she writes. "In this way, accepting the label can hamper your recovery."[18] Also, some days we may feel that work is all we have left. Unlike the unpredictable course of our disease or the complications it imposes on our personal relationships, paid work gives us a sense of control over a part of our lives that is uniquely our own.

I've thought longingly about applying for disability, but I can't conceive of not working at all. I would love to be able to work when I am able to and rest when I need to, but I suspect that even people without a chronic disease would like to have that freedom. As long as I can still put words on paper I'll keep working, but I hope I will have the good sense to know when I need to ask for help.

Steeling Ourselves for Appeals

Most initial SSDI applications for those of us with such illnesses as fibromyalgia and chronic fatigue syndrome are denied because we can still move our hands and arms and can stand, according to attorney Joshua Potter. We may file a request for reconsideration, which also is likely to be denied. Beyond that, we may request a hearing before an administrative law judge and, if that fails, we may seek review of our case by an appeals council. Our last resort is to file a lawsuit in the U.S. district court that serves our jurisdiction. The district court may agree with the administrative law judge or send the case back (remand it) for a new hearing.

Though each of our appeals must be filed within sixty days of a denial of benefits, SSA is under no time pressure to return a decision. Potter says it is not unusual for the entire process to take two years.[19]

Mary Ann Lyons received state disability payments for one year, after which she was expected to file for SSDI. Her application was denied, and she has filed an appeal. "The trouble with chronic fatigue syndrome is there's no way to test for it," Mary Ann says. "It's just what the patient reports to the doctor." A former social security claims representative herself, she understands but is not pleased by the process. Mary Ann is single and was working as a psychotherapist when she became sick. She is living on her savings while she tries to start a private practice counseling people with chronic disease.

Applying for disability would be daunting if we were well but when we are sick it can seem insurmountable. Half of the people who seek disability give up after the first or second denial, according to Miryam Williamson.[20] Ken Henderson was discouraged from even considering filing. "From what I've heard, if you tell the SSA you have fibromyalgia, they just grin and throw the form in the trash after you leave," he says. Persistence is one key to a successful decision, and careful preparation is another.

Keeping Detailed Records

To convince SSA of our disability, we need well-documented information about our medical condition and how it affects our ability to work. This means keeping a detailed account of how we feel and function on our worst days. We may note that we are unable to sit comfortably for more than a few minutes at a time, use a keyboard or write with a pen, or concentrate for extended periods. We also must educate our doctors about the disability process and the need for them to record specific information as well. According to Joshua Potter, our physician should document our ability to sit, stand, walk, lift, bend, and carry; note whether we can adhere to a regular work schedule and interact appropriately with others; and mention any behavioral factors, such as depression, associated with our disease. "A brief unsupported conclusion that the patient is unable to work will likely contribute to denial of benefits," Potter says.[21] However, he notes, the doctor should not offer an opinion about whether an individual is entitled to disability payments. "Disability is a legal construct, not a medical determination," according to Potter.[22] The SSA offers a guide for health professionals on providing medical evidence of disability for individuals with chronic fatigue syndrome. This fact sheet is one of many available on the SSA Office of Disability Web site; see the resources at the end of the book for more information.

Francie Moeller receives SSDI for fibromyalgia and degenerative disk disease because she was able to prove that an employer wouldn't be able to count on her to be at work. She says, "Employers have a right to know when you are going to work, and I can't tell them I'll be there at a certain time or on a certain day."

Using a Psychiatric Diagnosis

Certain chronic illnesses, such as fibromyalgia, are not included in the listing of impairments the SSA uses to evaluate medical conditions. In these cases, the SSA must determine that the individual's condition is of equal severity to an impairment that is on the list or that it prevents the individual from doing any work at all. Because of such difficulties, fewer than 10 percent of fibromyalgia patients meet the federal standard for disability, according to Connecticut rheumatologist Brian Peck.[23] Those of us with fibromyalgia and related illnesses may need to seek disability for a psychiatric condition, such as depression, that is associated with our disease and that is a listed impairment. Miryam Williamson notes that we shouldn't let our pride get in the way of accepting such a diagnosis.[24]

Seeking Legal Help

We can file an initial application for disability benefits with our local social security district office on our own, but we are well advised to seek legal counsel when our case is to be heard before an administrative law judge. We must have an attorney admitted to practice in U.S. district court if our case makes it this far. The National Organization of Social Security Claims Representatives refers individuals to attorneys who specialize in this work. The group's toll-free number is listed in the resources.

Attorneys who take disability cases generally receive a percentage of any award we receive. Disability payments, which range from $350 to $1,000 a month depending on the amount we have paid into the system, are retroactive to the sixth full month after our disability has begun, as determined by the SSA.[25] Two years after SSDI payments begin, we are eligible for Medicare, the federal health insurance program for disabled and retired persons. (Individuals without a substantial work history receive disability payments from the Supplemental Security Income [SSI] program and are also eligible for Medicaid.)

Because of the sometimes lengthy process, we are better off applying for disability as early as possible. But Angela waited for two years after multiple sclerosis forced her into retirement because she kept hoping she would go back to work. "When it became increasingly apparent that no one else believed I could go back to work, I applied for disability and got it right away," she says. Disability payments sustained her until she took a part-time consulting job.

Disability May Not Be Forever

Most of us want to have something productive to do. If we can't work full-time, we might seek part-time work to fill the void. However, most part-time jobs don't come with health insurance benefits. Further, if we are receiving SSDI, the income we earn from part-time work may jeopardize our disability payments and, ultimately, our Medicare benefits as well. According to the SSA, average earnings of $500 or more a month are considered "substantial," and our benefits may be discontinued if we have earned more than this amount for nine months in any five-year period.[26] The agency for which Angela works pays her $499.96 a month. Medicare benefits may continue for thirty-nine months after disability payments end.

SSA periodically reviews cases to see if an individual is still disabled. Our case will be reviewed after anywhere from six months to seven years depending on whether medical improvement is "expected," "possible," or "not expected," according to SSA guidelines.[27]

GOING IT ON OUR OWN

Many of us who can no longer maintain a 9-to-5 lifestyle but who want or need to be employed, end up working for ourselves. To do this, we have to have a product or a service we can sell, clients who want what we have to offer, and some financial support—savings, disability payments, or a spouse's income—to cushion us while we get our business off the ground. Sometimes we can fall back on the skills we've used for a lifetime, such as writing or counseling, to get us started. I negotiated a deal with my former employer to continue on a contract basis the work I had been doing for the company. The price of office equipment has come down in recent years, and it's possible to outfit a small home office, including a printer, computer, and fax machine, for less than $2,500.

For those of us who are less certain what we could do on our own, Miryam Williamson suggests we make a list of all the jobs we have held, including raising a family, and all the skills we have used in performing these jobs. "Turn off that tape running in the back of your mind that says, You can't do that," she writes. "No matter how much you have lost, there are still plenty of things you can do."[28]

"The Smartest Thing I Ever Did"

Miryam has been self-employed as a technical journalist since 1983. "Deciding to freelance was the smartest thing I ever did," she told me. "Setting up my office in my home was the second smartest thing. If I need a day off during the week, I can make it up on the weekend. You can't do that when you work for somebody else." Miryam admits, though, that she rarely gives in to the pain and fatigue of fibromyalgia. She gives herself plenty of lead time to complete assignments, and she knows that her clients are less concerned with how she gets the job done than with the fact that she finishes on time. She works in bed when she can't sit at her desk. Miryam never told any of her clients about her illness until she wrote about her experiences in *Fibromyalgia: A Comprehensive Approach*, which was published in 1996. "Now I've blown my cover," she told me.

My Own Worst Boss

Like Miryam, I work at home, and I am my own worst boss. Though I have the chance to nap every day, I reserve that option for only the worst of times. I feel that I need to keep my skills sharp and my clients happy. But my time is largely my own, and I can pick my son up at school or leave for a doctor's appointment as long as I get my work done. I enjoy being sought out for certain projects, and I am proud of the finished pieces I produce. Not having to look good or pretend to feel well frees energy I can put toward my work. Lack of distractions means I can focus on the task at hand.

Self-employment is not for everyone, however. With multiple clients to juggle, my workload and cash flow are unpredictable. This past year, I put many of my clients on hold while I worked on this book, and I wonder if they will be there when I am done. The quiet I cherish most days makes me feel lonely sometimes. I have no colleagues with whom to eat lunch or brainstorm creative ideas. I buy my own health insurance, and I pay a 15 percent self-employment tax. Finally, I'm aware that I might not be able to do this at all if I weren't married and didn't have a second income to fall back on.

Despite the drawbacks, however, I hope to be able to remain self-employed. I see it as the best chance I have to balance my need to be useful with my need to be healthy. Besides, I often think of that old joke about the circus worker who cleans up after the elephants. When a friend who hears him complaining about his job suggests that he look for another line of work, he replies, "What, and leave show business?" My place in the overall scheme of things may be small, but it's my own.

When Self-Employment Is Not a Choice

Miryam and I "chose" to work for ourselves, though I wonder if we would have made this choice had we not been ill. Ironically, I think that being sick gave me the courage I needed to start my own business. Had I felt physically able to continue working full-time, I likely would not have taken the risk. But others of us have very little choice at all. Too ill to work but unable to rely on another source of income, to qualify for disability, or to stretch our savings far enough, we may need to find something to fill the gap. Mary Ann Lyons was devastated when illness forced her to leave her job as a family therapist. As her health began to improve, and her money started to run out, she began slowly building a private practice. She held what she called a "women's day of renewal," which included guided meditations and a nature walk, and planned a workshop on coping with chronic disease. Afraid that if she takes another full-time job she'll get sick again, Mary Ann is using her own experience with chronic fatigue syndrome to help others learn how to take better care of themselves.

VOLUNTEERING OUR TIME

Useful work doesn't always come with a salary. Kathy Hammitt owns a business with her husband but she told me, "My passions are in a different place." She has long been involved with the Sjogren's Syndrome

Foundation and is currently serving a term as president. Kathy helped start local support groups, served as a contact person for prospective mothers with Sjogren's syndrome, and has testified before Congress on the need to fund research on chronic illnesses that predominantly strike women. She also is active in her children's schools. Her husband keeps the business running, and she contributes when she can.

Learning from Those We Serve

Like Kathy, many of us who have a chronic disease reach out to help others who are ill. We run support groups, field telephone calls, draft articles, and appeal to our legislators. Sometimes our volunteer activities help us develop new skills or lead to career opportunities. Angela's position on the board of directors of a nonprofit agency led to part-time employment. Other individuals I spoke to have become leading advocates for people with chronic fatigue syndrome, Lyme disease, and liver disease. We not only regain some sense of purpose for ourselves when we volunteer, we also learn from the people we serve. When I answer a call about Sjogren's syndrome, I am just as likely to come away with a new self-care tip or a better perspective on my disease as I am to pass along information to the person who called. A listing of organizations that welcome our help can be found in the resources at the end of this book.

RETHINKING WORK

Of all the issues I've dealt with since becoming ill, my relationship to my work has been the hardest to resolve. I agree wholeheartedly with such practical advice as that of author Cheri Register, who writes, "When illness makes it difficult to continue the work you have been doing, there are really two matters to resolve: 'What *must* I do to keep this illness from impoverishing me?' and 'What *can* I do now that I have physical limitations?' "[29]

But if the issue were simply one of how to make money and keep busy, that would be easy. The harder part for me, and I suspect for others, is to let go of the overriding sense that we are what we do. This attitude may impede our recovery because we're so busy doing, we have little time to take care of ourselves. Being sick in a world that prizes health and productivity can make us feel defective but it also gives us a rare opportunity to determine what is important in our lives, a topic we'll explore further in chapter 9.

I will always think of myself as a writer, but gradually I'm trying to let go of my need to be the best. Like Charlotte, the beloved spider in E. B. White's *Charlotte's Web*, I would like to be remembered for more than the work I do. "It is not often that someone comes along who is a true friend and a good writer," the narrator intones. "Charlotte was both."[30] Each of us needs to find our own healthy sense of balance concerning the role of work in our lives.

THE GIFT OF CHRONIC ILLNESS

In spite of illness . . . one can remain alive long past the usual
date of disintegration if one is unafraid of change, insatiable
in intellectual curiosity, interested in big things, and happy
in small ways.[1]
EDITH WHARTON

Chronic illness isn't a gift in the traditional sense of the word. We don't
want it or need it, it never fits, and we can't take it back. Only the most
idealistic among us would say that we are grateful to be sick. But once we
become ill, we can resent and reject the experience, or we can learn from
it. Just as an individual with a terminal illness may come to appreciate the
quality of the life he or she has left, those of us with a chronic disease often
find meaning in our pain. We discover hidden strengths, find a new sense
of direction, or adopt healthier habits.

I don't believe we become sick because we need to learn these
lessons. Most of us could lead perfectly happy lives without a chronic disease! But I do think that our illness, and the way we approach it, can teach
us much about ourselves. "When illness comes, it is, or can be, an invitation to move more deeply into our own lives," writes Dr. James S. Gordon.[2] In this final chapter, we'll explore how ill health can spur us to
spiritual and emotional growth and healthier living.

COMMON THREADS

Only a few of the people I interviewed hesitated when I asked what lesson their illness had taught them. I always prefaced my question by saying that I wasn't asking them to be a Pollyanna. Indeed, as Patricia A. Fennell says, "There isn't always a silver lining to chronic illness. Sometimes, there's just suffering." But she goes on to say that such suffering can transform us if it helps us to accept who we are, warts and all. And nearly everyone I spoke to had a story about the gift that illness has brought into their lives.

There are, of course, some common threads. Most of us have learned to slow the pace of our lives and to be more compassionate toward others. We've had to look deep inside ourselves and discover who we are apart from what we do. Some of us have found ways to share our experience, strength, and hope with others, by running support groups, writing books, or hosting on-line discussions. And all of us have made some wonderful friends along the way. To a person, we'd rather be healthy and have accomplished these things, but we've long ago stopped expecting miracles. In doing so, we have found the miraculous in our everyday lives.

SPIRITUAL GROWTH

"God becomes very personal when you're ill," Lexiann Grant-Snider told me. For many of us, chronic illness causes us to question our faith. We wonder if the God we believe in would cause such pain, or if illness is simply a random event. We reach outside ourselves, seeking solace and answers from a higher power, from spirit guides, or from the God we have prayed to since we were children.

Lexiann says that years of struggling with ill health have helped her meet God on a gut level. "I don't believe anymore that we always bring bad things on ourselves, or that an unloving, hellfire-and-brimstone type of God sends us woes as a punishment," Lexiann says. "But I do believe that everything that happens in our lives ultimately has a higher purpose for good, even if we never find out what that is." What are the gifts that Sjogren's syndrome and hepatitis have given her? "Learning how to reduce stress, time to write, time to spend with my dogs whom I love dearly and who love me, discovering my real friends, and certainty of hope in a spiritual life," Lexiann says.

The pain of undiagnosed interstitial cystitis following, as it did, her son's untimely death knocked Lenore to her knees. But she's not angry with God. Indeed, she believes that difficult times bring spiritual gifts. "I've been given the gifts of endurance, compassion, and a closer walk with God," Lenore told me. She seeks God less now that her pain has decreased. "There's a sort of complacency that sets in," she says.

Renewing Our Faith

A benevolent and loving God has been a part of my life since I was a small child, when my maternal grandmother did her best to instill in me the strong faith she had. But like Lenore, I became complacent for many years. Oh, I talked to God every day, but it was always to ask for something—a good mark on a test, a green light when I was in a hurry, an uneventful pregnancy and healthy child. Periodically, I attended one or another local church, but typically I went to church only on holidays for nearly fifteen years.

When I developed arthritis at age thirty-five and received a diagnosis of Sjogren's syndrome, I was scared. I didn't know what course my disease would take or how I would care for my son if I became seriously ill. An article in the local paper about a new church in the area caught my eye. I went the second Sunday that services were held, and I have been going ever since. The timing was right. I needed to hear the messages of hope and of faith that recalled for me my grandmother's words. I learned to pray in a different way, thanking God for how much he had already done to help me accept and overcome the limitations of chronic disease. Also, I made some wonderful friends, including the man I later married. Would I have gone back to church if I hadn't been ill? I can't really know but I suspect not. If my life had been humming along, I don't think I would have felt the need to reach out for help. Though I'm not glad I became sick, I am very grateful that my illness prompted me to explore and strengthen my faith.

EMOTIONAL DISCOVERY

Sometimes the profound sense of loss we experience as a result of chronic disease—including the loss of health, friends, work, and fun—

causes us to look inward. Relieved of the external trappings of employment and social status, we are left alone with ourselves. When we've never taken the time to know who we are, this can be a frightening proposition.

A Time for Taking Stock

"Middle age is a time for taking stock anyway, but fibromyalgia forced me to question myself," says Mireille. She had been divorced for many years, her children were grown, and she took early retirement because of her health. "I started looking at the big questions, like, Why am I here? and Where am I going?" she says. "It sounds pretty dramatic, but that was what I had to do." With the help of counseling, and time, Mireille made some important discoveries about herself. She learned she doesn't have to be a perfectionist to be a good person and that she doesn't have to explain her limitations to anyone unless she wants to. She's also less likely to try to change other people's habits or to have expectations of her friends and be disappointed when they don't meet them. "I wouldn't be feeling as well as I do emotionally if I hadn't gone through these growing pains," Mireille says. "I found out that my health may not be all right, but I am!"

Learning to Like Ourselves

Mireille's statement is fairly profound and one that many people, sick or well, would be hard-pressed to make. With all the talk of dysfunctional families, each of us seems to have some handicap that has stunted our self-esteem. Chronic illness gives us the opportunity to take stock of our lives and to discover what we like about ourselves. My self-esteem has always been based on being an achiever. If achievement becomes more difficult, I'd better have something to fall back on. That's the focus of much of the introspection and counseling I am doing now. Writing this book also has been part of that process. A very wise friend to whom I confided that I couldn't write a book on chronic illness until I had "all the answers" suggested that committing myself to this project might be just what I needed to do to find them. I knew something about how to look for doctors and research treatments before I started writing, but I understood little about how to accept myself as a person with a chronic disease. I'm glad to have learned that acceptance is a choice I can make for today.

Changing Our Approach to Life

If I'd met Jeri before she had lupus, I would have seen a very different person. Physically disabled from birth, her can-do spirit guided her through childhood and young adulthood. She had a great admiration for her own ability to overcome obstacles. But she couldn't overcome lupus; she had to learn to live with it. "This disease knocked me right on my butt," Jeri told me. "Then I had to rethink my whole philosophy. At age forty-five, I began to realize, Whoops, I got some of this life wrong."

Jeri was at once trying to deny, and to control, her disease. Instead, lupus was controlling her. She had to come up with some new solutions, and one of them was to stop fighting so hard. "I think the call for me was to find ways to not be so rigid," Jeri says. She watches birds from her kitchen window instead of hiking, and she always lets friends know that she might not be able to keep her plans. The Jeri I met was relaxed, generous, and open. "I like the things I've learned," she says. "I would like to be healthy again and still know them."

HEALTHIER HABITS

Perhaps it's just human nature that we have to get sick to become well. Our health is one of those things we pay little attention to as long as we have it. Getting Crohn's disease was a wake-up call for Bob. He ate what he wanted and had all but stopped exercising. When his waistline expanded, he bought bigger pants. But far from resenting the need to take better care of himself, Bob thinks this is the gift his illness has given him. "I feel more in control of my health," Bob says. "I'm eating less, and I'm eating better foods. I'm not carrying so much weight around my middle. I really had let myself go."

Workaholism was one of the poor health habits that Mary Ann Lyons had adopted. When chronic fatigue slowed her down, she was forced to look at the impact that obsessive work was having on her health and on her relationships. "If I hadn't gotten sick, I think I would have been stuck on the same old treadmill," Mary Ann says. But she didn't stop with work. She consulted a nutritionist about her diet, which was largely vegetarian but included sugar binges. She feels better now that she's more careful about what she puts in her mouth. "If I hadn't changed the way I was eating, I'm afraid to think how sick I would have been," she says.

People who become sick suddenly may be able to make the correlation between unhealthy habits and the symptoms of their disease. Those of us who have been sick for some time face a different challenge. We have a tendency to ignore symptoms that we attribute to our illness, thereby running the risk of missing a potentially serious complication or a new problem altogether. We don't need to call the doctor for every ache and pain, but we're aware enough of our own bodies to sense when something isn't right, and when that happens we should check it out.

SERVICE TO OTHERS

One of the women I spoke to while researching this book told me that having a chronic illness had caused her to become more compassionate toward others. I laughed when she added, "Of course, I'd rather be healthy and shallow." Somewhere along the line, someone probably told us that caring for others helps us forget our own problems. Though this may seem to be trite advice, many people say that it works. "Every day in my practice, I see people whom illness has made more generous," writes Dr. James Gordon. "Listen to the inner voice that urges you, in the midst of suffering, to reach out to someone else who is also suffering."[3] The challenge, of course, is to not do this so well that we neglect to take care of ourselves.

Focusing on Someone Else

Despite living most of her life with the pain of fibromyalgia, Dulce firmly believes that everything in life happens for a reason and her reason for having a chronic disease is to be able to help others. That's why she has committed so much of her time in recent years to researching her illness and sharing what she finds with anyone who can benefit from the information. In Internet discussion groups, she pays a good deal of attention to "newbies," those who sign on for the first time full of questions and fears. "I'm convinced that if I had someone like me twelve to fifteen years ago, I would not be in the shape I am today," Dulce says. "I would have known how to take better care of myself." By sharing her hard-won knowledge with others, Dulce says she also helps herself come to terms with her disease.

While I was writing this book, a number of people, including Dulce, told me they felt that the interviews I conducted were therapeutic. They found it helpful to talk about their experiences with chronic illness with someone who really was interested in knowing how they felt. Interestingly, and somewhat unexpectedly, I discovered there are far more similarities than differences among us. Women, as well as men, struggle with the impact that illness has on their careers. Men, as well as women, question their faith and rethink their identity. Those who are young worry about being good parents to their children, and those of us in middle age and beyond are concerned about being a burden to ours. As I shared my own story with the people I spoke to, I discovered some fears and strengths I hadn't been aware of until I gave voice to them. When we can reach out to others with whom we share an invisible but common bond, it doesn't really matter who is helping whom. Each of us is enriched by the experience.

A DELICATE BALANCE

Sometimes I'm a bit uneasy talking about how our lives have changed for the better since we've developed a chronic disease. We can all rationalize the worst of circumstances, but that doesn't make them good. Are we putting our heads in the sand when we find meaning in a life with chronic illness? I don't think so. After all, we could find that our lives are devoid of meaning and rail at our bad luck, but then we would be both sick *and* miserable. Those who seem most at peace with chronic disease have found the true gift of illness—the necessity, and the time, to find the good in life. The positive spin we put on our experiences is tinged with the reality of pain and disability, but however delicate the balance we have achieved, the foundation of our beliefs is strong and resilient.

Concentrating on the Small

Daniel impressed me with an almost folksy wisdom, born of the struggle to incorporate multiple sclerosis into his life. He used to commute to work by bus, an experience many of us would find inconvenient, at the least. But Daniel used the time to learn that there are some very decent people in this world.

"Sometimes I didn't get to the bus stop in time, but there was a woman who looked out for me," he says. "One time she made the bus driver back up a block to pick me up. Also, people who take buses are not in as much of a hurry as people who take trains. You have a chance to talk to them." Daniel's lifelong faith has helped him come to terms with his disease, but so too has his attitude that having a chronic illness means "it's time to concentrate on the small. There's a lot to appreciate in life that I might have missed had I not become ill," Daniel says, "like watching the change of seasons from a bus window."

Making Life Count

Kathy Hammitt told me that having Sjogren's syndrome has forced her to look at every day as if it were a gift. "I think most people whose lives change dramatically in a way that's unexpected are fortunate to learn early on to cherish life, especially to cherish their loved ones and to constantly think about their priorities," she says. Twice, Kathy has been told she might have cancer. "Not knowing if I'm going to be alive in a year or two makes me wonder, 'Is this what I want to be doing with my time?' So it makes me live my life much better." When Kathy parcels out her limited energy, she gives the bulk of it to her family and to her work with the Sjogren's Syndrome Foundation. "My having a chronic illness has brought my family much closer together," Kathy says. "Many people don't get that early nudge to make life count."

Figuring Out What's Important

Angela's identity was formed before she had multiple sclerosis. When the disease changed her life, she had to change with it. "Having a chronic illness makes you stop and assess what's important in your life and what isn't," she told me. "You realize that what's important in life isn't work, and it isn't things. What's important in life are people, those you care about and those who care about you, and the relationships you have with them. It just took awhile for me to figure that out."

Angela looked inward to decide what she wanted to be involved in while she's alive, and how she wanted to be remembered when she's gone. "You only go around once in life, and you have to do what you can to make that life a little better for everyone around you," she says. "That's the way I live my life now."

Living in balance with our disease is really a very practical way to live. Pam, Pam's daughter, and Pam's mother all have fibromyalgia, so Pam doesn't have the luxury of having a negative outlook on life. "Loss of energy means I've lost the ability to feel rage over silly things, and I've learned the value of empathy and understanding," she says. "By moving more slowly, I see the good in most people, and the humor in everyday life."

THE GIFT OF KNOWING OURSELVES

Looking at the comments I made to those I interviewed, I noted that even I, a cynical journalist who is sometimes passionately attached to her negative opinions, have found gifts in chronic disease. The opportunity to write this book tops the list. I'd like to think that I would have written a book about something else, but I can't know that for certain. I have been told that successful writers write about what they know. Certainly, I know the pain, fear, and frustration of living with chronic disease, but I also know the joy of working toward a dream. For this I am grateful and somewhat in awe.

Also, I am thankful for the friends I have made, many of whose stories are told in these pages. They help me laugh when humor escapes me but they never make light of my confusion or my pain. Their generosity of spirit, particularly in sharing some very painful and intimate details of their lives, is an inspiration to me. In the conclusion, I'm happy to be able to share some of the key lessons they taught me.

Finally, and most importantly, I've been enriched by what ill health has taught me about myself. Like many of us, I try to push past my disease, thereby making my symptoms and my mood much worse. "I'll sleep when I'm old," I say cavalierly to those who suggest that I work too hard. What a gift it is to learn that it is not only okay but also imperative for me to strike a delicate balance between my need to be productive and my need to take care of myself. I suspect I might have missed this lesson had I not become sick. I have a sign over my computer that reads, "As soon as the rush is over, I'm going to have a nervous breakdown. I worked for it, I owe it to myself, and nobody is going to deprive me of it." That's the old Susan. The one who is slowly coming to grips with chronic disease owes herself a nice vacation. I'm certain I'll take it, just as soon as my work is done!

CONCLUSION

Many of my friends think the work I do is depressing. Professionally, I write about the health care needs of homeless people. Though I am saddened by their situation, when I have the privilege of interviewing people who are homeless, I am touched by their humility, honesty, and sense of hope. This past year, I chose to spend much of my time chronicling the lives of those who live every day with chronic disease. Along the way, I spoke at length to three dozen of my fellow patients. But my research was far from dispiriting. Once again, I was struck by the sense of compassion and strength with which people face adversity. As I laughed with these individuals and learned from them, I began to feel layers of isolation and denial peel away. Since this has been an intensely personal journey, I'd like to share with you in these final pages what these warm and generous men and women taught me about living successfully with chronic disease. Ultimately, I learned much about myself.

DOING THINGS THE HARD WAY

I've often been accused of doing things the hard way. Call it stubbornness or curiosity, but when people give me advice, I want to know how they acquired their wisdom. Indeed, I've read many articles and books about chronic illness that profess much the same message contained within these pages: namely, that we need to stop looking for someone or something else to make us better and start learning to take care of ourselves. Yet, without knowing the struggles that come between misfortune and acceptance, I've always rejected such guidance as being too pat or not based in reality. Now I know that is simply not the case. The individuals I spoke with have come to accept life with a chronic disease slowly and sometimes grudgingly. No one I talked to told me not to worry or to "just relax." But the women and men I came to know also made it abundantly clear that when we adopt a woe-is-me attitude, we are doomed to spend the rest of our days both sick *and* miserable. Seen in that light, learning to live effectively in spite of chronic illness seems like very practical advice.

LESSONS FROM THE FRONT

The overall message I received from the people I interviewed is that while chronic illness changes our lives forever, such change is not necessarily bad. More specifically, many of the people I spoke to left me with a particular message of hope, strength, or acceptance. These lessons from the front have changed me forever.

From Sally, I learned that I need to accept that I am a person with a chronic disease (several, in fact). This seems like such a simple lesson, yet it's one that has been so difficult for me to learn. I don't want to be deficient or defective; I want to be just like everybody else. But Sally taught me that my struggles to pass as healthy were consuming valuable energy that I could better use to take care of myself. Her advice didn't come out of a book; she has lived for more than half her life with chronic fatigue syndrome, and she only recently acknowledged that she has a real illness herself. When I am tempted to deny reality, I think of Sally's story about the color of the sky. No matter how hard I might wish for the sky to be purple, she says, the sky will still be blue and I will be unhappy about it. Sally sees my striving and knows the toll it takes on me. Though we have only just met, she has become one of my closest friends.

Angela taught me that attitude is everything. She disputed the working title of this book, *It's Not All in Your Head*, because she said that attitudinal change *is* in our heads. Until I spoke to her at length, I was afraid she was going to try to convince me that if only I were happier, I would be healthier. But Angela has some significant disabilities, the result of living with multiple sclerosis for sixteen years. Even she has days when she's unhappy. But if she dwells on these days, Angela told me, she has more of them. Plus, she can't afford to be gloomy around the people who help her to remain as independent as possible. Her advice to me clearly was hard-won. On my bad days, I can picture Angela curled up with her cat and a pot of tea and know that this too shall pass.

I have always attempted to use my intellect, and more recently, my growing faith, to try to understand the world around me. Friends and family know that I am always asking, Why? Daniel impressed on me the fact that I can't know everything. He is a scientist who has researched diseases similar to multiple sclerosis, which he has. Still, he accepts the fact that he will never fully understand the disease process. Daniel also is an Orthodox Jew, the son and brother of rabbis. Though his religion gives him comfort, he acknowledges that it doesn't help him understand why he has this disease. Neither formal education nor religious training have helped Daniel coexist peacefully with multiple sclerosis; that comes from his willingness to accept the uncertainties in his life. Ironically, by letting go of my need to find *the* answer, I receive the insight I'm seeking.

From Pam, I have a very clear sense of the need to laugh. Not that much in her life has been funny. Pam, her mother, and her teenage daughter all have fibromyalgia, and her daughter has to live with relatives to accommodate her need for special schooling. But Pam finds the humorous in everyday life. She delights in the absurd, and much of what we experience with chronic illness falls into that category. I know that Pam's laughter may hide some well-deserved tears, but I can delight in her sense of humor, and in my own, when I need to shed my serious approach to life.

I like Jeri's description of herself as a can-do person. But I am equally struck by the humility with which she accepts the fact that she can't conquer lupus. Like Jeri, I think of myself as a take-charge individual. How could I write this book while living with chronic illness myself, nurturing a new marriage, raising a teenage son, and running a business? No problem, I told wary family and friends. But I, too, have been humbled. The strain of meeting my various commitments has left me exhausted more days that not. I have learned intimately, in a way that no book or research article could teach me, about the impact of stress on chronic disease. By driving myself as hard as I could, I have finally come up against my limits. Slowly, I have begun to respect them.

I have started to treat myself to simple pleasures, and to simplify my life. Rediscovering a favorite hobby, I have stocked my bookshelves with novels. Reading helps me unwind at the end of a long day. For the first time in my life, I am allowing myself to wear my hair both straight and short because it eases the morning routine that sometimes wears me out. Realizing that my stamina is limited, I am far less likely to let petty annoyances disturb me. When I'm not feeling well, I have a network of support on which to draw. My friends don't allow me to wallow in pity, but they understand my frustrations and fears, and they offer healthy, useful advice.

THE JOURNEY CONTINUES

I mentioned in the preface that both my son and my best friend were sick the year I wrote this book. My son, thankfully, recovered nicely after having his tonsils out. Though my friend still has undiagnosed symptoms, she has begun to feel better, in part because when she parcels out her energy, she spends some of it on herself. Learning to live successfully with a chronic disease is really nothing more or less than learning to live a balanced life. When our expectations and desires are out of line with our abilities and our resources, we are bound to feel poorly. Accepting ourselves as full and worthwhile human beings who happen to have a chronic disease is not the end of our journey. Rather, self-acceptance and self-care are the beginning of a healthier and more fulfilling existence. I will miss working on this book, but I am anxious to begin the next chapter of my life.

NOTES

CHAPTER 1

1. Camille A. Jones and Leroy Nyberg, "Epidemiology of Interstitial Cystitis," *Urology*, vol. 49, no. 5A (May 1997), 2–9.
2. Don L. Goldenberg, *Chronic Illness and Uncertainty: A Personal and Professional Guide to Poorly Understood Syndromes* (Newton Lower Falls, MA: Dorset, 1996), 15.
3. Daniel J. Clauw, "The Pathogenesis of Chronic Pain and Fatigue Syndromes, with Special Reference to Fibromyalgia," *Medical Hypotheses* 44 (1995), 369–378.
4. Carol S. Burckhardt and A. Bjelle, "Perceived Control: A Comparison of Women with Fibromyalgia, Rheumatoid Arthritis, and Systemic Lupus Erythematosus Using a Swedish Version of the Rheumatology Attitudes Index," *Scandinavian Journal of Rheumatology*, vol. 25, no. 5 (1996), 300–306.
5. S. Bombardieri, et al., "Diagnostic Criteria for Sjogren's Syndrome," *Proceedings of the Fourth International Symposium on Sjogren's Syn-*

drome in Tokyo, Japan, 11–13 August 1993 (New York: Kugler, 1994), 73–76.

6. Beverly M. Calkins, "Inflammatory Bowel Diseases," in *Digestive Diseases in the United States: Epidemiology and Impact,* ed. James E. Everhart (Bethesda, MD: National Institutes of Health, May 1994), 519.

7. Patricia A. Fennell, "The Four Progressive Stages of the CFS Experience: A Coping Tool for Patients," *Journal of Chronic Fatigue Syndrome,* vol. 1, no. 3/4 (1995), 69–79.

8. Hillary Johnson, *Osler's Web: Inside the Labyrinth of the Chronic Fatigue Syndrome Epidemic* (New York: Crown, 1996).

9. Leonard A. Jason, et al., "Politics, Science, and the Emergence of a New Disease: The Case of Chronic Fatigue Syndrome," *American Psychologist,* vol. 52, no. 9 (Sept. 1997), 001–0011.

10. Clauw, 372.

11. Linda Hanner, *Healing Wounded Doctor–Patient Relationships* (Delano, MN: Kashan, 1995), 125–126.

12. Fennell, 70.

13. Hanner, 43.

14. Hanner, 27.

15. Myasthenia gravis is an autoimmune disorder in which the body's immune system attacks and gradually destroys receptors in muscles that are responsible for picking up nerve impulses. The affected muscles fail to respond or respond only weakly to nerve impulses, and as a result they become weak and tire easily. The muscles of the eyes, face, throat, and limbs are most commonly affected.

16. Hanner, 5–6.

17. Goldenberg, 22.

18. Charles B. Clayman, ed., *American Medical Association Home Medical Encyclopedia* (New York: Random House, 1989), 763.

19. Hanner, 143.

20. Hanner, 3.

21. "Lyme Disease Cases Rose 41% in 1996, CDC Says," *Palm Beach Post,* 13 June 1997, 4A.

22. "Lyme Borreliosis in Europe," *Risk: Epidemiology,* on-line posting, European Union Concerted Action on Lyme Borreliosis, Internet, 15 Aug. 1997. Available: http://www.dis.strath.ac.uk/vie/LymeEU/risk-epid.htm

23. Goldenberg, 87.

24. *Fibromyalgia Syndrome and Chronic Fatigue Syndrome Index and Glossary* (Tucson, AZ: Health Information Network, 1996), 2–19.
25. Goldenberg, 100.
26. Muhammad B. Yunus, "Fibromyalgia Syndrome: Clinical Features and Spectrum," *Journal of Musculoskeletal Pain*, vol. 2, no. 3 (1994), 5–21.
27. Clauw.
28. Mary Anne Dunkin, "Fibromyalgia: Syndrome of the '90s," *Arthritis Today*, vol. 11, no. 5 (Sept.–Oct. 1997), 40–47.
29. Clauw.
30. Michael E. Ruane, "Gulf War Syndrome Lacks Scientific Proof, Medical Panel Finds," *Knight-Ridder/Tribune News Service*, 9 Oct. 1996, 1009K5428.
31. Daniel J. Clauw, M. D., assistant professor of medicine, Georgetown University Medical Center, testimony before the Subcommittee on Human Resources and Intergovernmental Relations of the House Committee on Government Reform and Oversight, regarding illnesses and diseases reported by veterans who served in the Persian Gulf War, 28 March 1996.
32. Yunus.
33. Dr. Muhammad Yunus, personal communication with Miryam Williamson, 21 Sept. 1997.
34. Daniel J. Clauw and Paul Katz, "The Overlap between Fibromyalgia and Inflammatory Rheumatic Disease: When and Why Does It Occur?" *Journal of Clinical Rheumatology*, vol. 1, no. 6 (Dec. 1995), 335–341.

CHAPTER 2

1. Daniel J. Clauw, M. D., assistant professor of medicine, Georgetown University Medical Center, testimony before the Subcommittee on Human Resources and Intergovernmental Relations of the House Committee on Government Reform and Oversight, regarding illnesses and diseases reported by veterans who served in the Persian Gulf War, 28 March 1996.
2. See, for example, James S. Gordon, *Manifesto for a New Medicine: Your Guide to Healing Partnerships and the Wise Use of Alternative Therapies* (New York: Addison-Wesley, 1996), 23; and Don L. Goldenberg, *Chronic Illness and Uncertainty: A Personal and Professional Guide to Poorly Understood Syndromes* (Newton Lower Falls, MA: Dorset, 1996), 112–113.
3. Gordon, 24.

4. Patricia A. Fennell, "CFS Sociocultural Influences and Trauma: Clinical Considerations," *Journal of Chronic Fatigue Syndrome*, vol. 1, no. 3/4 (1995), 159–173.

5. D. Buchwald, et al., "Race and Ethnicity in Patients with Chronic Fatigue," *Journal of Chronic Fatigue Syndrome*, vol. 2, no. 1 (1996), 53–66.

6. Linda Hanner, *Healing Wounded Doctor–Patient Relationships* (Delano, MN: Kashan, 1995), 126.

7. Hanner, 125.

8. Fennell, 167.

9. Agency for Health Care Policy and Research, *Depression in Primary Care: Volume 1. Detection and Diagnosis* (Rockville, MD: Agency for Health Care Policy and Research, 1993), 55.

10. Daniel J. Clauw, "Fibromyalgia: More than Just a Musculoskeletal Disease," *American Family Physician*, vol. 52, no. 3 (1 Sept. 1995), 843–851.

11. Susan Swedo and Henrietta Leonard, *It's Not All in Your Head* (New York: HarperCollins, 1996), 101.

12. Hanner, 138.

13. "Chronic Fatigue Syndrome: A Modern Medical Mystery," *Newsweek*, 12 Nov. 1990, 62–70.

14. Hanner, 142.

15. Katrina Berne, "Life on Seven Brain Cells a Day: Neurocognitive Problems and Coping Skills in CFIDS/FMS," on-line posting, Sapient Health Network, Internet, 25 Jan. 1997. Available: http://www.shn.net

16. A. T. Slotkoff and Daniel J. Clauw, "Fibromyalgia: When Thinking Is Impaired," *Journal of Musculoskeletal Medicine*, vol. 13, no. 9 (Sept. 1996), 32–36.

17. Goldenberg, 66.

18. "Systemic Lupus Erythematosus," *Primer on Rheumatic Diseases*, 10th ed. (Atlanta, GA: Arthritis Foundation, 1993), 106–116.

19. Hanner, 133–134.

20. Gordon, 103.

21. Andrew Weil, *Spontaneous Healing: How to Discover and Enhance Your Body's Natural Ability to Maintain and Heal Itself* (New York: Fawcett Columbine, 1995), 98.

22. Mark J. Pellegrino, *Fibromyalgia: Managing the Pain* (Columbus, OH: Anadem, 1993), 68.

23. Thomas Romano, "Medico-Legal Aspects of Post-Traumatic Fibromyalgia and Myofascial Pain," *Health Points*, vol. 2, no. 2 (Fountain Hills, AZ: TyH Publications, Spring 1997), 1–3.

24. "New Studies Show Fetal Cells May Trigger Autoimmune Disease," *The Moisture Seekers Newsletter,* vol. 15, no. 6 (Jericho, NY: Sjogren's Syndrome Foundation, Sept. 1997), 1.
25. Walter B. Cannon, *The Wisdom of the Body* (New York: Norton, 1926).
26. Hans Selye, *The Stress of Life* (New York: McGraw-Hill, 1956).
27. Selye, 1.
28. Selye, 36.
29. Gordon, 98.
30. Selye, 38.
31. Selye, 169.
32. Gordon, 98. See also Devin Starlanyl and Mary Ellen Copeland, *Fibromyalgia and Chronic Myofascial Pain Syndrome: A Survival Manual* (Oakland, CA: New Harbinger, 1996), 140.
33. Selye, 169.
34. Daniel J. Clauw, "The Pathogenesis of Chronic Pain and Fatigue Syndromes, with Special Reference to Fibromyalgia," *Medical Hypotheses* 44 (1995), 369–378.
35. Fennell, 163.
36. Norman Cousins, *Anatomy of an Illness as Perceived by the Patient* (New York: Norton, 1979), 34.
37. Cousins, 86.
38. Goldenberg, 1. See also Jeff Kane, *Be Sick Well: A Healthy Approach to Chronic Illness* (Oakland, CA: New Harbinger, 1991), 13.

CHAPTER 3

1. Marion Crook, *My Body: Women Speak Out about Their Health Care* (New York: Insight Books-Plenum, 1995), 131.
2. Linda Hanner, *Healing Wounded Doctor–Patient Relationships* (Delano, MN: Kashan, 1995), 12.
3. Timothy B. McCall, *Examining Your Doctor: A Patient's Guide to Avoiding Harmful Medical Care* (Secaucus, NJ: Citadel–Carol, 1995), 9.
4. Hanner, 14.
5. Hanner, 22.
6. James S. Gordon, *Manifesto for a New Medicine: Your Guide to Healing Partnerships and the Wise Use of Alternative Therapies* (New York: Addison-Wesley, 1996), 26.
7. Gordon, 28.

8. Don L. Goldenberg, *Chronic Illness and Uncertainty: A Personal and Professional Guide to Poorly Understood Syndromes* (Newton Lower Falls, MA: Dorset, 1996), 36.

9. Hanner, 21.

10. John Caher, "Woman Battles Two Foes: Disease and Her Insurer," *Albany (NY) Times Union*, 26 May 1997, A1.

11. McCall, p. 59, and Hanner, 69.

12. Elizabeth Lee Vliet, *Screaming to Be Heard: Hormonal Connections Women Suspect . . . and Doctors Ignore* (New York: Evans, 1995), 363.

13. Hanner, 40.

14. Andrew Weil, *Spontaneous Healing: How to Discover and Enhance Your Body's Natural Ability to Maintain and Heal Itself* (New York: Fawcett Columbine, 1995), 59.

15. McCall, 17.

16. Gordon, 87.

17. McCall, 52.

18. McCall, 298.

19. Crook, 142.

20. Hanner, 165.

21. McCall, 284.

22. McCall, 16.

23. McCall, 108.

24. Weil, 249.

25. McCall, 300.

26. McCall, 295.

27. McCall, 10.

28. Gordon, 295.

29. Susan Milstrey Wells, "Exploring the Promises and Pitfalls of Managed Care," *Access*, vol. 7, no. 1 (Delmar, NY: National Resource Center on Homelessness and Mental Illness, Mar. 1995), 1–5; Susan Milstrey Wells, "An Introduction to Managed Behavioral Health Care: Implications for Public Mental Health and Substance Abuse Services," unpublished article, 1996; and McCall, 32–40.

CHAPTER 4

1. Norman Cousins, *Anatomy of an Illness as Perceived by the Patient* (New York: Norton, 1979), 62.

2. Miryam Ehrlich Williamson, *Fibromyalgia: A Comprehensive Approach* (New York: Walker, 1996), 42.
3. Robert Bennett and Glenn McCain, "Coping Successfully with Fibromyalgia," *Patient Care*, 15 March 1995, 29–45.
4. Williamson, 42.
5. Bennett and McCain.
6. "Focus On . . . Rheumatoid Arthritis," *Medical Sciences Bulletin* (Levittown, PA: Pharmaceutical Information Associates, Dec. 1994). On-line posting, Pharmaceutical Information Network, Internet, 16 May 1997. Available: http://www.pharminfo.com/pubs/msb/rheumart.html
7. Stephen Barrett, "Quackery in the Media," in *The Health Robbers: A Close Look at Quackery in America*, eds. Stephen Barrett and William Jarvis (Buffalo, NY: Prometheus, 1993), 448.
8. James S. Gordon, *Manifesto for a New Medicine: Your Guide to Healing Partnerships and the Wise Use of Alternative Therapies* (New York: Addison-Wesley, 1996), 196.
9. Cousins, 123.
10. William Jarvis and Stephen Barrett, "How Quackery Sells," in Barrett and Jarvis, 11–12.
11. Gina Kolata, "On Fringes of Health Care, Untested Therapies Thrive," *New York Times*, 17 June 1996, A1.
12. Gordon, 69, and Barrett and Jarvis, 355.
13. Jeff Kane, *Be Sick Well: A Healthy Approach to Chronic Illness* (Oakland, CA: New Harbinger, 1991), 86.
14. David M. Eisenberg, et al., "Trends in Alternative Medicine Use in the United States, 1990–1997," *The Journal of the American Medical Association*, vol. 280, no. 18 (11 Nov. 1998), 1569–1575.
15. David Eisenberg, et al., "Unconventional Medicine in the United States: Prevalence, Costs, and Patterns of Use," *New England Journal of Medicine*, vol. 328, no. 4 (28 Jan. 1993), 246–252.
16. George Howe Colt and Joe McNally, "See Me, Feel Me, Touch Me, Heal Me: Medical Doctors Who Incorporate Alternative Medicine," *Life*, vol. 19, no. 10 (Sept. 1996), 34–44.
17. For more information about the Oxford Health Plan alternative medicine program, see the Oxford Web site at http://www.oxhp.com
18. Edward W. Campion, "Why Unconventional Medicine?" *New England Journal of Medicine*, vol. 328, no. 4 (28 Jan. 1993), 282–283.
19. Gordon, 22.
20. William T. Jarvis and Stephen Barrett, "How Quackery Sells," in Barrett and Jarvis, 21.

21. Timothy B. McCall, *Examining Your Doctor: A Patient's Guide to Avoiding Harmful Medical Care* (Secaucus, NJ: Citadel–Carol, 1995), 67.
22. Charles B. Inlander, Lowell S. Levin, and Ed Weiner, *Medicine on Trial* (New York: Prentice Hall, 1988), 154.
23. Marion Crook, *My Body: Women Speak Out about Their Health Care* (New York: Insight Books-Plenum, 1995), 149.
24. William T. Jarvis and Stephen Barrett, "How Quackery Sells," in Barrett and Jarvis, 13.
25. Gordon, 104–105.
26. Sarah Van Boven, "Giving Infants a Helping Hand," *Newsweek Special Edition: Your Child,* Spring/Summer 1997, 45.
27. Bill Moyers, *Healing and the Mind* (New York: Doubleday, 1993), 87–88.
28. David Spiegel, et al., "Effect of Psychosocial Treatment on Survival of Patients with Metastatic Breast Cancer," *Lancet,* 14 Oct. 1989, 888–891.
29. Gordon, 222–223.
30. Gordon, 271.
31. Gina Kolata, "In Quests Outside Mainstream, Medical Projects Rewrite Rules," *New York Times,* 18 June 1996, A1.
32. Robert L. Park and Ursula Goodenough, "Buying Snake Oil with Tax Dollars," *New York Times,* 3 Jan. 1996, A15.
33. Crook, 106.
34. H. K. Beecher, "The Powerful Placebo," *Journal of the American Medical Association* 159 (1955), 1602–1606.
35. Cousins, 56.
36. Cousins, 49–50.
37. Eisenberg, et al., 1998, 1993.
38. Cynthia K. Lefton, "Fen/Phen: What's the Fuss All About?" On-line posting, Sapient Health Network, Internet, 15 Apr. 1997. Available: http://www.shn.net
39. Heidi M. Connolly, et al., "Valvular Heart Disease Associated with Fenfluramine–Phentermine," *New England Journal of Medicine,* vol. 337, no. 9 (28 Aug. 1997), 581–588.
40. Lauran Neergaard, "Two Popular Diet Drugs Pulled from Shelves," *Albany (NY) Times Union,* 16 Sept. 1997, A1.
41. Kolata, "On Fringes of Health Care."
42. Geoffrey Cowley, "Herbal Warning," *Newsweek,* 6 May 1996, 60–67.
43. Cowley.
44. Gordon, 160.
45. Cowley.

46. Stuart L. Nightingale, "Update on EMS and L-tryptophan," *Journal of the American Medical Association*, vol. 268, no. 14 (14 Oct. 1992), 1828.
47. Gordon, 159.
48. McCall, 289–291.

CHAPTER 5

1. "Homeopathy," *Harvard Women's Health Watch*, vol. 4, no. 5 (Jan. 1997), 2–3.
2. James S. Gordon, *Manifesto for a New Medicine: Your Guide to Healing Partnerships and the Wise Use of Alternative Therapies* (New York: Addison-Wesley, 1996), 181.
3. *Harvard Women's Health Watch*.
4. Stephen Barrett and William Jarvis, eds., *The Health Robbers: A Close Look at Quackery in America* (Buffalo, NY: Prometheus, 1993), 360–361.
5. *Harvard Women's Health Watch*.
6. Beth Anne Serepca, "Interview with Tiffany Field, Ph.D.," *Massage* 63 (Sept.–Oct. 1996), 44–48.
7. Sarah Van Boven, "Giving Infants a Helping Hand," *Newsweek Special Edition: Your Child*, Spring–Summer 1997, 45.
8. David M. Eisenberg, et al., "Trends in Alternative Medicine Use in the United States, 1990–1997," *The Journal of the American Medical Association*, vol. 280, no. 18 (11 Nov. 1998), 1569–1575.
9. Van Boven.
10. Serepca, 46.
11. Janet Macrae, *Therapeutic Touch: A Practical Guide* (New York: Knopf, 1987), 3.
12. Joe Maxwell, "Nursing's New Age?" *Christianity Today*, vol. 40, no. 2 (5 Feb. 1996), 96–99.
13. Maxwell.
14. National Institutes of Health, *Alternative Medicine: Expanding Medical Horizons* (Bethesda, MD: National Institutes of Health, Dec. 1994), 146.
15. Lori Oliwenstein, "Craving a Cure," *Arthritis Today*, vol. 10, no. 3 (May–June 1996), 33–39.
16. Oliwenstein.
17. Jeff Kane, *Be Sick Well: A Healthy Approach to Chronic Illness* (Oakland, CA: New Harbinger, 1991), 103.
18. Elaine Gloria Gottschall, *Breaking the Vicious Cycle: Intestinal Health through Diet* (Kirkton, Ontario: Kirkton, 1994).

19. Roy L. Swank and Barbara Brewer Dugan, *The Multiple Sclerosis Diet Book: A Low-Fat Diet for the Treatment of MS* (New York: Doubleday, 1987).
20. Barry Sears and Bill Lawren, *Enter the Zone: A Dietary Road Map to Lose Weight Permanently, Reset Your Genetic Code, Prevent Disease, Achieve Maximum Physical Performance* (New York: HarperCollins, 1995).
21. Gordon, 43.
22. Gordon, 154.
23. Kane, 102.
24. Varro E. Tyler, *Tyler's Honest Herbal: A Sensible Guide to the Use of Herbs and Related Remedies* (Binghamton, NY: Haworth Press, 1999).
25. Norman Cousins, *Anatomy of an Illness as Perceived by the Patient* (New York: Norton, 1979), 84.
26. Peter Doskoch, "Happily Ever Laughter," *Psychology Today*, vol. 29, no. 4 (July–August 1996), 32–35.
27. Mark J. Pellegrino, *Laugh at Your Muscles: A Light Look at Fibromyalgia* (Columbus, OH: Anadem, 1995), 12.
28. "A Funny Thing Happened on the Way to Recovery," *Journal of the American Medical Association,* vol. 267, no. 13 (1 Apr. 1992), 1856–1857.
29. Doskoch.
30. Claudia Wallis, "Faith and Healing: Can Prayer, Faith, and Spirituality Really Improve Your Physical Health? A Growing and Surprising Body of Scientific Evidence Says They Can," *Time*, vol. 147, no. 26 (24 June 1996), 58–62.
31. "Family Physician Survey Topline Report," (Radner, PA: John Templeton Foundation, Oct. 1996).
32. Wallis.
33. Wallis.
34. George Howe Colt and Joe McNally, "See Me, Feel Me, Touch Me, Heal Me: Medical Doctors Who Incorporate Alternative Medicine," *Life*, vol. 19, no. 10 (Sept. 1996), 34–44.
35. Herbert Benson, *The Relaxation Response* (New York: Morrow, 1975).
36. Wallis.
37. Gordon, 106.
38. Kane, 8.
39. Gordon, 106.
40. Gordon, 118.
41. National Institutes of Health, 22.

42. Edward B. Blanchard, et al., "Direction of Temperature Control in the Thermal Biofeedback Treatment of Vascular Headache," *Applied Psychophysiology and Biofeedback* (in press).
43. Gordon, 128–129.
44. Kane, 127.
45. "Tai Chi," *Harvard Women's Health Watch,* vol. 4, no. 3 (Nov. 1996), 4.
46. David D. Burns, *Feeling Good: The New Mood Therapy* (New York: Morrow, 1980), 12.
47. Jane E. Brody, "Changing Thinking to Change Emotions," *New York Times,* 21 Aug. 1996, C9.
48. Lucia Capacchione, *The Picture of Health: Healing Your Life with Art* (Van Nuys, CA: Newcastle, 1996).
49. Bardi Koodrin, "Drawing Out the Spirit," in *We Laughed, We Cried: Life with Fibromyalgia,* eds. Kit Gardiser and Kathleen Kerry (Palo Alto, CA: KMK Associates, 1995), 91–103.

CHAPTER 6

1. Andrew Weil, *Spontaneous Healing: How to Discover and Enhance Your Body's Natural Ability to Maintain and Heal Itself* (New York: Fawcett Columbine, 1995), 103.
2. Jeff Kane, *Be Sick Well: A Healthy Approach to Chronic Illness* (Oakland, CA: New Harbinger, 1991), 3.
3. James S. Gordon, *Manifesto for a New Medicine: Your Guide to Healing Partnerships and the Wise Use of Alternative Therapies* (New York: Addison-Wesley, 1996), 286.
4. Elisabeth Kübler-Ross, *On Death and Dying* (New York: Macmillan, 1969).
5. Patricia A. Fennell, "CFS Sociocultural Influences and Trauma: Clinical Considerations," *Journal of Chronic Fatigue Syndrome,* vol. 1, no. 3/4 (1995), 159–173.
6. Patricia A. Fennell, "The Four Progressive Stages of the CFS Experience: A Coping Tool for Patients," *Journal of Chronic Fatigue Syndrome,* vol. 1, no. 3/4 (1995), 69–79.
7. Fennell, "The Four Progressive Stages," 73–79.
8. Kübler-Ross, 39.
9. Fennell, "The Four Progressive Stages," 70.
10. Norman Cousins, *Anatomy of an Illness as Perceived by the Patient* (New York: Norton, 1979), 152.

11. Ogden Nash, *There's Always Another Windmill* (Boston: Little, Brown, 1967), 103–104.
12. Fennell, "CFS Sociocultural Influences."
13. Elaine Showalter, *Hystories: Hysterical Epidemics and Modern Culture* (New York: Columbia University, 1997).
14. Hillary Johnson, *Osler's Web: Inside the Labyrinth of the Chronic Fatigue Syndrome Epidemic* (New York: Crown, 1996).
15. DEPRESSION Awareness, Recognition, and Treatment (D/ART) Program, *Depression: What Every Woman Should Know* (Rockville, MD: National Institute of Mental Health), 1.
16. Kane, 61.
17. Dianne Witter, "When You're among Friends," *Arthritis Today*, vol. 10, no. 5 (Sept.–Oct. 1996), 41–46.
18. Sheldon Cohen, et al., "Social Ties and Susceptibility to the Common Cold," *Journal of the American Medical Association*, vol. 277 (1997), 1940–1944.
19. Albert Schweitzer, *Out of My Life and Thought* (New York: Holt, Rinehart, and Winston, 1949), 194.
20. Jan Bresnick, "The Secret Weapon against America's Biggest Health Threats," *Prevention*, vol. 46, no. 12 (Dec. 1994), 84–88.
21. Bresnick.
22. Bresnick.
23. "Finding Medical Help Online," *Consumer Reports*, vol. 62, no. 2 (Feb. 1997), 27–31.
24. Newsgroup Watch, *Yahoo! Internet Life*, vol. 3, no. 2 (Feb. 1997). Online posting, *Yahoo!*, 30 Sept. 1997. *Internet Life*, Internet. Available: http://www.zdnet.com/yil/content/mag/9702/news9702.html
25. Lynne Lamberg, "Patients Go On-Line for Support," *American Medical News*, vol. 39, no. 13 (1 Apr. 1996), 16–19.
26. Michael Parrish, "On-Line Medical Advice," *American Health*, Oct. 1996, 39–41.
27. *Consumer Reports*, 31.
28. Naomi Freundlich, "Trading in the Couch: Brief Therapy," *Harvard Health Letter*, vol. 19, no. 12 (Oct. 1994), 1.
29. Kane, 14, 35.
30. Kane, 42.
31. Weil, 251–252.
32. Kane, 155.

CHAPTER 7

1. Jeff Kane, *Be Sick Well: A Healthy Approach to Chronic Illness* (Oakland, CA: New Harbinger, 1991), 60.
2. Alan Booth and David R. Johnson, "Declining Health and Marital Quality," *Journal of Marriage and the Family* 56 (Feb. 1994), 218–223.
3. Linda Welsh and Marian Betancourt, *Chronic Illness and the Family: A Guide for Living Every Day* (Holbrook, MA: Adams Media, 1996), 94.
4. Miryam Ehrlich Williamson, *Fibromyalgia: A Comprehensive Approach* (New York: Walker, 1996), 133.
5. Welsh and Betancourt, 117.
6. Welsh and Betancourt, 116.
7. Welsh and Betancourt, 161.
8. Williamson, 139.
9. Williamson, 140–141.
10. Welsh and Betancourt, 189.
11. Welsh and Betancourt, 154.
12. Kane, 66.
13. Welsh and Betancourt, 68.
14. Welsh and Betancourt, 68.
15. Welsh and Betancourt, 71.
16. Katherine M. Hammitt, "Statement of Sjogren's Syndrome Foundation Scheduled for Presentation on June 12, 1991, before the Task Force on Opportunities for Research on Women's Health, National Institutes of Health," 6.
17. Elaine K. Harris, ed., *The Sjogren's Syndrome Handbook* (Jericho, NY: Sjogren's Syndrome Foundation, 1989), 135.
18. Williamson, 146–147.
19. Williamson, 145.
20. Kane, 71.
21. Welsh and Betancourt, 49–50.

CHAPTER 8

1. Robert M. Bennett, et al., "Group Treatment of Fibromyalgia: A Six-Month Outpatient Program," *The Journal of Rheumatology*, vol. 23, no. 3 (1996), 521–528.
2. Miryam Ehrlich Williamson, *Fibromyalgia: A Comprehensive Approach* (New York: Walker, 1996), 153.

3. Studs Terkel, *Working: People Talk about What They Do All Day and How They Feel about What They Do* (New York: Pantheon, 1974), 422–424.

4. With acknowledgment to Dr. Meyer Friedman and Dr. Ray Rosenman, whose book *Type A Behavior and Your Heart* (New York: Knopf, 1974) first described the hard-driving Type A *behavior* that makes certain individuals susceptible to heart attacks, and its more relaxed counterpart, Type B. The concept of a Type B *body* is my own.

5. Cheri Register, *Living with Chronic Illness: Days of Patience and Passion* (New York: Macmillan, 1987), 95.

6. U.S. Equal Employment Opportunity Commission and U.S. Department of Justice, *Americans with Disabilities Act Handbook* (Washington, DC: U.S. Equal Employment Opportunity Commission and U.S. Department of Justice, Dec. 1991), I–25, I–27.

7. U.S. Equal Employment Commission and U.S. Department of Justice. I–41.

8. U.S. Equal Employment Commission and U.S. Department of Justice. I–44.

9. U.S. Equal Employment Commission and U.S. Department of Justice. I–38.

10. L. M. Sixel, "Skepticism Greets Some Disabilities," *Albany (NY) Times Union,* 15 July 1996, C2.

11. U.S. Department of Justice, "Myths and Facts about the Americans with Disabilities Act," On-line posting, U.S. Department of Justice ADA Home Page, Internet, 27 June 1997. Available: http://www.usdoj.gov/crt/ada/pubs/mythfct.txt

12. U.S. Department of Justice, "Myths and Facts."

13. U.S. Equal Employment Opportunity Commission and U.S. Department of Justice, I–64, I–70.

14. Janice Strubbe Wittenberg, *The Rebellious Body: Reclaim Your Life from Environmental Illness or Chronic Fatigue Syndrome* (New York: Insight Books-Plenum, 1996), 193.

15. Jon Hamilton, "FMS and Disability: Finding the Best Path to Compensation," On-line posting, Sapient Health Network, Internet, 10 Jan. 1997. Available: http://www.shn.net

16. Social Security Administration, *Disability* (Baltimore, MD: Social Security Administration, May 1996), 3.

17. Joshua W. Potter, "Helping Fibromyalgia Patients Obtain Social Security Benefits," *Journal of Musculoskeletal Medicine,* vol. 9, no. 9 (Sept. 1992), 65–74.

18. Wittenberg, 193.
19. Potter, 65–74.
20. Williamson, 162.
21. Potter, 65–74.
22. Jon Hamilton, "Fibro and Disability: Making a Claim Takes an Arsenal of Weapons," on-line posting, Sapient Health Network, Internet, 7 Jan. 1997. Available: http://www.shn.net
23. Jon Hamilton, "FMS and Disability: Finding the Best Path to Compensation," on-line posting.
24. Williamson, 163.
25. Potter.
26. Social Security Administration, 17.
27. Social Security Administration, 16.
28. Williamson, 159.
29. Register, 104.
30. E. B. White, *Charlotte's Web* (New York: HarperCollins, 1952), 184.

CHAPTER 9

1 Edith Wharton, *A Backward Glance* (New York: Appleton-Century, 1934), vii.
2 James S. Gordon, *Manifesto for a New Medicine: Your Guide to Healing Partnerships and the Wise Use of Alternative Therapies* (New York: Addison-Wesley, 1996), 299.
3. Gordon, 297.

GLOSSARY

Italicized terms in definitions are also defined in this glossary.

ADRENAL GLANDS   Small, triangular-shaped endocrine (hormone-producing) glands that sit atop the kidneys and secrete hormones directly into the bloodstream to regulate metabolism and to control the body's *stress* response.

AMERICANS WITH DISABILITIES ACT (ADA)   Comprehensive legislation passed in 1990 that prohibits discrimination against individuals with disabilities in employment, state and local government services, and public accommodations. Title I of the ADA allows individuals who are disabled to seek *reasonable accommodations* that allow them to meet the essential functions of their job.

AMITRIPTYLINE   An inexpensive and widely used antidepressant medication that increases levels of *serotonin* and is frequently effective in treating *fibromyalgia* and related disorders.

ARTHRITIS   More than one hundred different diseases that cause pain, swelling, and limited movement in joints and *connective tissues* throughout the body. Types of arthritis include osteoarthritis, a degenerative joint disease, as well as the *autoimmune diseases* rheumatoid arthritis, *Sjogren's syndrome*, and *lupus*.

AUTOIMMUNE DISEASE   A disorder in which the body mistakes its own cells as foreign invaders. Examples include *Sjogren's syndrome, lupus*, and rheumatoid arthritis.

AUTONOMIC NERVOUS SYSTEM   That part of the nervous system that controls involuntary or automatic functions, such as heart rate and breathing. The autonomic nervous system is made up of the *sympathetic* and the parasympathetic branches.

BRAIN FOG   A term used by people to describe the *cognitive dysfunction* that may accompany their disease.

BIOFEEDBACK   A relaxation technique in which individuals are taught to recognize and alter changes in their *autonomic nervous system* when offered some type of perceptible recording of the change, such as use of a high-pitched sound or electronic graph.

CAPITATION   Literally "by the head," a method for paying a health care provider a fixed price per person served for a specified time period and for a defined range of services. *Managed care* organizations rely, to a greater or lesser degree, on capitation financing.

CARPAL TUNNEL SYNDROME   Numbness and pain in the hands and forearms that results from pressure on the median nerve (one of the main nerves of the arm) as it passes through a gap in the wrist into the palm of the hand. Possible causes include a repetitive strain injury or *arthritis*.

CATECHOLAMINES   A group of chemical messengers like epinephrine (adrenaline) or norepinephrine that help control the body's *autonomic nervous system*. People with such illnesses as *fibromyalgia* and *chronic fatigue syndrome* may not produce sufficient catecholamines to protect them from pain and fatigue after exercise.

COGNITIVE BEHAVIORAL THERAPY   A behavioral technique that helps individuals recognize and change negative thought patterns that create unhealthy emotions.

COGNITIVE DYSFUNCTION   Symptoms including memory loss, forget-fulness, poor concentration, and confusion that affect many individuals with chronic disease. Multiple factors may contribute to cognitive dysfunction, including mood disorders, medications, fatigue, pain, and sleep disturbances. See *brain fog*.

CONNECTIVE TISSUE   The material that holds the body together. Connective tissue diseases, those that are marked by inflammation in the muscles, joints, and skin, often accompany illnesses like *Sjogren's syndrome*.

CHRONIC FATIGUE SYNDROME   A *syndrome* characterized by debilitating fatigue of unknown cause. To be diagnosed with chronic fatigue syndrome, patients must have severe, unexplained fatigue that lasts for six or more consecutive months and is not relieved by rest, along with at least four of eight additional symptoms, including sore throat, muscle pain, and impaired memory or concentration problems.

COMPUTERIZED AXIAL TOMOGRAPHY (CAT) SCAN   A diagnostic technique that combines the use of a computer and X rays to produce clear, cross-sectional images of the tissue being examined.

DISEASE   A disorder, such as *multiple sclerosis* or *lupus*, that is marked by measurable, physiological abnormalities.

DYSREGULATION SPECTRUM SYNDROME (DSS)   As defined by Dr. Muhammad B. Yunus, an overlapping group of illnesses that includes *fibromyalgia, chronic fatigue syndrome, irritable bowel syndrome*, and migraine headaches, among others. Dr. Yunus believes these illnesses are likely to result from abnormalities in the body's neurological, hormonal, and immune system functions.

EOSINOPHILIA MYALGIA SYNDROME (EMS)   A rare disorder characterized by severe muscle pain and an increase in eosinophils, a type of white blood cell, that caused illness and death in individuals who took a contaminated batch of *L-tryptophan*.

FEN/PHEN   An *off-label use* of the prescription diet drugs fenfluramine and phentermine used by some to treat such illnesses as *fibromyalgia* and *chronic fatigue syndrome*. In July 1997, fenfluramine was voluntarily withdrawn from the market when it was revealed that fen/phen causes heart valve damage.

FIBROMYALGIA   A *syndrome* marked by diffuse musculoskeletal pain and fatigue. Patients must have widespread pain in all four quadrants of the body for a minimum of three months and at least eleven of eighteen specified tender points to be diagnosed with *fibromyalgia*.

FIGHT-OR-FLIGHT RESPONSE   Activity on the part of the *sympathetic nervous system* that prepares animals to protect themselves against a perceived threat. During the fight-or-flight response, blood pressure, heart rate, and muscle tension go up, and the digestive and immune systems are depressed.

FLAMING   The *Internet* equivalent of a nasty argument.

GASTROENTEROLOGIST   A physician trained in the management of digestive system disorders.

GATEKEEPER   In a *managed care* organization, an individual (typically a patient's primary care physician) whose job it is to determine whether referrals for laboratory tests or specialist care are medically necessary.

HEALTH MAINTENANCE ORGANIZATION (HMO)   A type of *managed care* organization that provides comprehensive services to a defined group of subscribers for a fixed fee (see *capitation*). HMOs employ their own providers, contract with independent or group practice providers, or offer a combination of these plans.

HOMEOPATHY   A system of medicine developed by nineteenth-century German physician Samuel Hahnemann based on the belief that "like cures like." Homeopaths use substances that produce similar disease symptoms in healthy people to provoke the body's immune response. Homeopathic remedies are so dilute that it is highly unlikely that even a single molecule of the original substance remains in the pill or liquid.

5-HYDROXYTRYPTOPHAN (5-HTP)   A breakdown product of the amino acid *L-tryptophan* used by some to treat fatigue.

INFLAMMATORY BOWEL DISEASE   An inflammatory disorder of the small or large intestine marked by abdominal pain, diarrhea, and weight loss. Inflammatory bowel disorders include Crohn's disease, ulcerative colitis, and ulcerative proctitis.

INTERNET   A worldwide network of computers that communicate with one another.

INTERSTITIAL CYSTITIS   A chronic inflammation of the bladder. Urgency, frequency, and pain are the principal symptoms of this disorder.

IRRITABLE BOWEL SYNDROME   A disorder marked by abdominal pain and intermittent constipation and diarrhea. Irritable bowel often accompanies such illnesses as *fibromyalgia*.

L-TRYPTOPHAN   An amino acid that is a precursor of the brain chemical *serotonin*. Used by many individuals with chronic disease to treat fatigue, L-tryptophan was recalled by the U.S. Food and Drug Administration when a contaminated batch caused an outbreak of *eosinophilia myalgia syndrome*.

LUPUS   See *systemic lupus erythematosus*.

LYME DISEASE   An infectious, tick-transmitted disorder that results in flu-like symptoms and joint inflammation. First identified in Old Lyme, Connecticut, in 1975, Lyme disease is especially prevalent in the New England and mid-Atlantic states.

LYMPHOCYTES   A type of white blood cell that protects the body by killing viruses and bacteria. In patients with *Sjogren's syndrome*, lymphocytes invade and destroy body tissues.

LYMPHOMA   A cancer of the lymph glands that develops in fewer than 5 percent of *Sjogren's syndrome* patients.

MAILING LIST   A group of messages on a particular topic maintained by a list owner and delivered to subscribers by E-mail. Numerous mailing lists focus on health-related topics.

MAGNETIC RESONANCE IMAGING (MRI)   The use of powerful magnetic fields and radio waves to provide high-quality, cross-sectional images of organs and structures within the body.

MANAGED CARE   A method for organizing and delivering health care that seeks to control costs and utilization through such methods as *capitation* financing, prior approval of tests and specialist referrals, and the use of provider networks.

MULTIPLE SCLEROSIS   A progressive disease of the central nervous system that destroys scattered patches of myelin (the protective covering of nerve fibers) in the brain and spinal cord. Symptoms range from numbness and tingling to incontinence and paralysis.

NEWSGROUP   A virtual bulletin board accessed via the *Internet* that is open to anyone who wants to participate. Many newsgroups focus on health-related issues.

NEUROTRANSMITTER   A chemical messenger that transmits nerve impulses in the body.

NIGHTSHADES   More than seventeen hundred species of trees, shrubs, and herbs in the genus *Solanum,* including such common foods as bell peppers, eggplants, potatoes, and tomatoes. The theory that nightshades cause arthritis has not been proven.

NONSTEROIDAL ANTI-INFLAMMATORY DRUGS (NSAIDs)   Over-the-counter and prescription medications used to control pain and inflammation.

OFF-LABEL USE   The use of a drug for purposes other than that for which it was developed.

OTOLARYNGOLOGIST   An ear, nose, and throat specialist.

PAIN   A sensation that results from stimulation of special sensory nerve endings following injury or caused by disease. Such adjectives as stabbing, throbbing, dull, burning, gnawing, and aching are used to describe pain.

PLACEBO   From the Latin verb meaning "I shall please," an inert substance once given more to please patients than to benefit them. In modern usage, placebos are used as controls in studies of new medications.

PREDNISONE   A corticosteroid drug, similar to the corticosteroid hormones produced by the body's *adrenal glands,* used to reduce inflammation and suppress an overactive immune system.

REASONABLE ACCOMMODATION   According to the *ADA,* any modification or adjustment to the job application process or work environment that enables an individual with a disability to perform the essential functions of a position for which he or she is qualified.

RELAXATION RESPONSE   As described by Dr. Herbert Benson, a specific set of physiological changes that occur when a person repeats a word, sound, or phrase, often called a "mantra," and passively disregards intrusive thoughts. Dr. Benson demonstrated that during the relaxation response, heart rate, respiration, and brain waves slow down, muscles relax, and the production of stress-related hormones diminishes, thereby countering the *fight-or-flight response.*

RHEUMATOLOGIST   A doctor who specializes in treating arthritis and other disorders of the joints, muscles, and *connective tissues.*

SELECTIVE SEROTONIN REUPTAKE INHIBITORS (SSRIs)   A class of antidepressant medication that inhibits the reuptake of *serotonin* and allows it to exert a longer-lasting effect.

SEROTONIN   A *neurotransmitter* that controls sleep states, consciousness and moods. Serum levels of serotonin are low in some people with *fibromyalgia.*

SJOGREN'S SYNDROME   An *autoimmune disease* marked by inflammation and eventual destruction of the body's exocrine (moisture-producing) glands. Symptoms include dry eyes, dry mouth, and vaginal dryness.

SOCIAL SECURITY DISABILITY INSURANCE (SSDI)   Benefits paid by the Social Security Administration (SSA) to disabled individuals based on prior work experience. The SSA definition of disability is strict and sometimes difficult for individuals with such illnesses as *fibromyalgia* and *chronic fatigue syndrome* to meet.

SOMATIZATION DISORDER   A psychiatric condition marked by bodily complaints for which no physical cause can be found. Some scientists and physicians believe that *fibromyalgia* and *chronic fatigue syndrome* are primarily somatization disorders, though recent research indicates distinct physiologic abnormalities in individuals with these illnesses.

SPAMMING   Sending messages indiscriminately to multiple *Internet* sites, especially *newsgroups.* Often, spammers have a product or service to sell.

STRESS   As defined by Dr. Hans Selye, the nonspecific response of the body to any demand. Dr. Selye differentiated between stress, the resulting condition, and stressor, the causative agent.

SUBSTANCE P   A peripheral *neurotransmitter* that initiates a pain signal following injury. Some people with *fibromyalgia* have low levels of substance P in their spinal fluid.

SYMPATHETIC NERVOUS SYSTEM   That part of the *autonomic nervous system* that prepares the body for action by activating the *fight-or-flight response.*

SYNDROME   A disorder, like *fibromyalgia* or *chronic fatigue syndrome,* that is characterized by a collection of symptoms patients report to their doctor and physical signs that the physician can see. Syndromes may cause illness in the absence of any observable *disease.*

SYSTEMIC LUPUS ERYTHEMATOSUS   An inflammatory, *autoimmune disease* that affects various parts of the body, including the skin, joints, blood, and kidneys.

TAI CHI CHUAN   A Chinese system of meditative exercises. Tai chi is considered a martial art, yet its movements are smooth and flowing, inspired by animals in nature.

THERAPEUTIC TOUCH   A therapy derived from the ancient practice of laying-on of hands and based on the assumption that there is a universal life energy that sustains all living organisms. By holding their hands several inches from an individual's body, practitioners believe they can assess and balance a patient's energy field.

WORLD WIDE WEB   The newest and fastest growing section of the *Internet* that features a scattered collection of pages, with both text and graphics, developed by individuals, institutions, and commercial firms. Web pages typically contain links to other relevant sites.

INDIVIDUALS PROFILED

Individuals with first names only are using pseudonyms. All other names are real. Individuals are listed in order of their appearance in the text.

EILEEN, 49, is single. She has interstitial cystitis and lupus. In search of a cause for her chronic bladder problems, Eileen agreed to have a hysterectomy, even though she has never had children. Therapy helped Eileen confront her losses. She struggled with her decision to retire after twenty-eight years of teaching fourth grade. Today, Eileen heads a local interstitial cystitis support group and writes educational plays for children.

KEN HENDERSON, 50, is married and the father of two grown children. He has fibromyalgia. Ken had a difficult time getting a diagnosis. Along the way, he had a healthy gallbladder removed and was sent to a psychiatric hospital. He lost his job for using too much sick time and had to cash in his retirement. If he had it to do over, Ken would put less effort into securing a diagnosis and more energy into getting well.

KATHY HAMMITT, 44,   is married and the mother of two school-aged children. She has Sjogren's syndrome. Chronic illness has given Kathy a reason to make life count. She focuses her energy on her work with the Sjogren's Syndrome Foundation and on her children. Kathy has been a support group leader and lobbyist for the foundation, and she is the current president. She wants to be seen as more than her illness.

DANIEL, 46,   is married and has two school-aged sons. He has multiple sclerosis. Daniel was diagnosed on a routine physical, and his disease has progressed rapidly. As a scientist, he had researched similar disorders. Daniel relies on a strong faith to understand who he is apart from his illness. He sprinkles his conversations with liberal doses of self-deprecating wit.

LINDA WEBB, 45,   is married and has two grown daughters. She has ulcerative proctitis. Fear kept Linda from seeking help for her symptoms for nearly a year. As an adopted child, she wishes she knew more about her birth parents' medical history. Linda finds it difficult to handle the travel that her job for a retail trade association requires. She would like to start a computer consulting business.

SALLY, 31,   is married and feels that she is not well enough to have children. She has chronic fatigue syndrome. Sally has been ill since she was 13, but only received a diagnosis eight years ago. She spent ten years finishing a doctorate in clinical psychology, despite ongoing illness. Sally and her husband, GARY, have struggled with her inability to earn an income. Gary heads an E-mail discussion group for spouses of people with chronic fatigue syndrome.

MIRYAM EHRLICH WILLIAMSON, 60,   is married and the mother of three grown children. She has fibromyalgia. Miryam was diagnosed at age 57, but she remembers being in pain as young as age 5. When she couldn't find a good book on fibromyalgia, she decided to write one. Miryam's book, *Fibromyalgia: A Comprehensive Approach*, was published in 1996. Her biggest regret is that she was sick when her children were young and couldn't explain why.

KELLY, 33,   is married and the mother of two school-aged children. She has lupus. Kelly had seemingly unconnected symptoms for years until exposure to ultraviolet radiation in a tanning booth brought her disease to the fore. She struggles with the impact that lupus and the medications she takes for it have on her physical appearance. Kelly's children are sensitive to her needs, but she worries they may be growing up too fast.

JERI, 52,   is married and the mother of four grown children. She has lupus. Jeri was born with a physical disability that gave her a can-do attitude toward life. She had to rethink her approach when she discovered that she couldn't conquer lupus. Jeri has struggled with the physical and emotional isolation that chronic illness imposes. When she has "overwhelming feelings of wellness," Jeri and her husband celebrate together.

DULCE, 63,   is married and the mother of two grown children. She has fibromyalgia. Even though she only recently received a diagnosis, Dulce believes she has had fibromyalgia most of her life. She spent many years covering up physical awkwardness and cognitive difficulties, mostly by learning to laugh at herself. Dulce helps others by gathering and disseminating information on fibromyalgia.

MIREILLE, 51,   is divorced, and her two children are grown. She has fibromyalgia. When illness forced her to retire from work at about the same time her children left home, Mireille experienced a profound sense of loss. She embarked on what she calls a "spiritual quest" to reinvent herself. Today, Mireille practices tai chi, sets clear limits, and uses humor to diffuse potentially embarrassing or awkward situations.

PAM, 39,   is married and the mother of a teenage daughter. Pam, her mother, and her daughter all have fibromyalgia, and Pam feels that that has opened up lines of communication among them. Her daughter lives with relatives so she can attend a school that is responsive to her health problems. Pam denied her own symptoms for many years. Her illness has taught her to find the humor in everyday life.

LEXIANN GRANT-SNIDER, 39,   is married, and she considers the Norwegian Elkhounds she raises to be her children. Lexiann has Sjogren's syndrome and hepatitis. When she went for years with no diagnosis, despite traveling to see numerous specialists, Lexiann sank into a deep depression. Her dogs provide company and a second income; Lexiann writes for national publications aimed at canine enthusiasts. Her husband, JIM SNIDER, and her best friend, DENISE TUCKER, share their thoughts about loving someone with a chronic disease.

JOAN O'BRIEN-SINGER, 57,   is married, and both she and her husband have Lyme disease. Joan had trouble securing a diagnosis and has been refused the long-term antibiotic treatment she believes she needs. But she says that when life gives you Lyme, you should make "Lyme-aide." She is cohost of a Lyme disease discussion group on America Online. Joan is seeking reasonable accommodations to allow her to continue working as a substance abuse counselor.

LOIS ARIAS, 45,   is married and the mother of a preschool-aged son. She has interstitial cystitis. Lois's family and friends have been a tremendous support to her, and she in turn reaches out to others. She is a former coleader of an interstitial cystitis support group on America Online. Lois found relief from her symptoms using an experimental antibiotic treatment.

LENORE, 44,   is married, and her only son died at the age of 20. She has interstitial cystitis. Lenore believes that childhood incest contributed to her bladder problems, because she involuntarily clenches her pelvic muscles under stress. She has had no symptoms of her illness since she prayed with a friend. Lenore believes that the pain of her son's death and her own illness have made her a more compassionate person.

WENDY HAY, 34,   is married and has two school-aged sons. She has multiple sclerosis and clinical depression. Wendy says that every day there is a minute when she wishes her multiple sclerosis would go away. A local support group has been her lifeline. Wendy has explained her disease in age-appropriate ways to both her boys. One of the first and most important lessons she learned from being sick was how to say no.

BOB, 34,   is married and the father of two school-aged children. He has Crohn's disease. Bob feels that his disease was a warning sign that he wasn't taking good care of himself. He finds that relaxation and exercise improve how he feels. Bob has been open with his employer about his diagnosis but he doesn't dwell on his symptoms at work. He has explained to his children that he is "a little bit sick all the time."

ANGELA, 49,   is married and is childless by choice. She has multiple sclerosis. Angela defined herself by her work as a disability advocate and was devastated when her own disability forced her to retire. She became an active volunteer. Angela's adoptive mother denied that Angela was ill and refused to be seen with her. Angela faces life with a positive attitude that is hard won but sincere.

MARY ANN LYONS, 47,   is single. She has chronic fatigue syndrome. Mary Ann is a licensed marriage and family therapist, and when illness forced her to leave full-time work she discovered that she had focused on her job to the exclusion of her personal life. She has used diet, art therapy, Chinese herbs, acupuncture, and imagery in search of better health. Mary Ann is developing workshops on personal growth and healing.

RESOURCES

CHAPTER 1

National Organizations

Contact these groups for information, local support groups, and volunteer opportunities.

Arthritis Foundation
National Office
1330 West Peachtree Street
Atlanta, GA 30309
(800) 283-7800/(404) 872-7100
http://www.arthritis.org

Crohn's & Colitis Foundation of
America, Inc.
386 Park Avenue South, 17th floor
New York, NY 10016-8804
(800) 932-2423/(212) 685-3440
Fax: (212) 779-4098
http://www.ccfa.org

The CFIDS Association of America,
Inc.
P.O. Box 220398
Charlotte, NC 28222-0398
(800) 442-3437/(704) 365-2343
Fax: (704) 365-9755
info@cfids.org
http://www.cfids.org

Fibromyalgia Alliance of America
P.O. Box 21990
Columbus, OH 43221-0990
(888) 717-6711/(614) 457-4222
Fax: (614) 457-2729

Fibromyalgia Network
P.O. Box 31750
Tucson, AZ 85751-1750
(800) 853-2929/(520) 290-5508
Fax: (520) 290-5550
http://www.fmnetnews.com

Interstitial Cystitis Association
51 Monroe Street, Suite 1402
Rockville, MD 20850
(800) 435-7422/(301) 610-5300
Fax: (301) 610-5308
http://www.ichelp.org

Lupus Foundation of America
1300 Piccard Drive, Suite 200
Rockville, MD 20850
(800) 558-0121/(301) 670-9292
Fax: (301) 670-9486
http://www.lupus.org

Lyme Disease Foundation
One Financial Plaza
Hartford, CT 06103
(800) 886-5963/(860) 525-2000
lymefnd@aol.com

Multiple Sclerosis Foundation, Inc.
6350 North Andrews Avenue
Fort Lauderdale, FL 33309-2130
(800) 441-7055/(954) 776-6805
Fax: (954) 938-8708
msfacts@juno.com
http://www.msfacts.org

National Chronic Fatigue Syndrome
and Fibromyalgia Association
P.O. Box 18426
Kansas City, MO 64133
(816) 313-2000
Fax: (816) 524-6782

National Multiple Sclerosis Society
733 Third Avenue, 6th floor
New York, NY 10017-3288
(800) 344-4867/(212) 986-3240
Fax: (212) 986-7981
Nat@nmss.org
http://www.nmss.org

Sjogren's Syndrome Foundation, Inc.
366 N. Broadway, Suite PH2W
Jericho, NY 11753
(800) 475-6473/(516) 933-6365
Fax: (516) 933-6368
http://www.sjogrens.org

CHAPTER 4

To view an updated list of alternative
medicine courses taught at U.S. medical schools, visit the Rosenthal Center
for Complementary and Alternative
Medicine World Wide Web site at:
http://cpmcnet.columbia.edu/dept
/rosenthal/guide.html

To purchase a copy of the National
Center for Complementary and
Alternative Medicine Report,
*Alternative Medicine: Expanding Medical
Horizons*, contact:
Superintendent of Documents
P.O. Box 371954
Pittsburgh, PA 15250-7954
(202) 512-1800/Fax: (202) 512-2250
Order document #017-040-00537-7 for
$29 ($36.25 foreign).

CHAPTER 5

To purchase a general information packet for $7 that includes the *Directory of Homeopathic Practitioners*, contact:
The National Center for Homeopathy
801 North Fairfax Street, Suite 306
Alexandria, VA 22314
(703) 548-7790
Fax: (703) 548-7792
nchinfo@igc.apc.org
To search the directory on-line, see:
http://www.homeopathic.org

For more information on massage, contact:
American Massage Therapy Association
820 Davis Street, Suite 100
Evanston, IL 60201-4444
(847) 864-0123
Fax: (847) 864-1178
http://www.amtamassage.org

International Massage Association
3000 Connecticut Avenue, Suite 308
Washington, DC 20008
(202) 387-6555
Fax: (202) 332-0051
http://www.imagroup.com

For more information on cognitive behavioral therapy, contact:

The Beck Institute for Cognitive Therapy and Research
GSB Building
City Line and Belmont Avenues
Suite 700
Bala Cynwyd, PA 19004-1610
(610) 664-3020
Fax: (610) 664-4437
beckinst@gim.net
http://www.beckinstitute.org

For more information on art therapy, contact:
American Art Therapy Association, Inc.
1202 Allanson Road
Mundelein, IL 60060
(847) 949-6064
Fax: (847) 566-4580
estygariii@aol.com
http://www.louisville.edu/groups/aata-www

To locate a health-related newsgroup:
DejaNews
http://www.dejanews.com

To locate a public mailing list:
L-Soft International
http://www.lsoft.com/lists/listref.html

CHAPTER 6

Journals on-line.
Journal of the American Medical Association
http://www.jama.ama-assn.org

New England Journal of Medicine
http://www.nejm.org

World Wide Web search engines:
Yahoo!®
http://www.yahoo.com

Alta Vista™
http://www.altavista.com
Lycos®
http://www.lycos.com

Other World Wide Web sites of interest:
healthfinder®
http://www.healthfinder.gov
Maintained by the U.S. government; includes links to selected on-line publications, clearinghouses,

databases, Web sites, self-help groups, government agencies, and nonprofit organizations.

Health*touch*®
http://www.healthtouch.com
Includes drug information, health organizations and government agencies, and information about specific health topics, diseases, and illnesses.

National Library of Medicine
http://www.nlm.nih.gov
Features free access to MEDLINE, the National Library of Medicine's database of more than 3,800 biomedical journals.

National Organization for Rare Disorders, Inc.
http://www.rarediseases.org
Learn about rare disorders, link to other health-related Web sites, and find support groups.

InteliHealth™
http://www.intelihealth.com
Health information from Johns Hopkins, including breaking news, disease-specific information, and free e-mail subscriptions.

WebMD^SM *Health*
http://my.webmd.com

Information on specific health topics, including fibromyalgia, chronic fatigue syndrome, and women's health. *WebMD* makes aggregate information about subscribers available to advertisers, but does not divulge individual data included in voluntary health profiles.

About.com™
http://home.about.com/health
Features a network of sites on specific health conditions led by "expert guides."

For information on caregiver support, contact:
Well Spouse Foundation
610 Lexington Avenue, Suite 814
New York, NY 10022-6005
(800) 838-0879/(212) 644-1241
Fax: (212) 644-1338
wellspouse@aol.com
http://www.wellspouse.org

National Family Caregivers Association
9621 East Bexhill Drive
Kensington, MD 20895-3104
(800) 896-3650/(301) 942-6430
Fax: (301) 942-2302
info@nfcacares.org

CHAPTER 8

For information on regulations, technical assistance, and enforcement for title I (employment) of the Americans with Disabilities Act, contact:
Equal Employment Opportunity Commission
1801 L Street NW
Washington, DC 20507
(800) 669-4000 (voice)
(800) 669-6820 (TDD)
http://www.eeoc.gov

To order a single copy of the *Americans with Disabilities Handbook* (about 400 pages) free of charge:
(800) 669-3362 (voice)
(800) 800-3302 (TDD)
For more information, see the U.S. Department of Justice ADA Home Page: http://www.usdoj.gov/crt/ada/adahom1.htm

For more information about the Social Security Disability Insurance program, contact:
The Social Security Administration
(800) 772-1213 (voice)
(800) 325-0778 (TTY)
http://www.ssa.gov/odhome
The chronic fatigue fact sheet is SSA Pub. 64-063/ICN 953800.

To find a private attorney specializing in Social Security claims law, contact:
The National Organization of Social Security Claims Representatives
(800) 431-2804

INDEX

Social Security Disability Insurance (SSDI)
(*cont.*)
legal help, seeking, 210–211
proof needed for, 207–208
psychiatric diagnosis, 210
record keeping, 209–210
Societal stigma, 47
Somatization disorder, defined, 253
Spamming, 153–154, 253
Specialization in health care, 17
Spiegel, David
breast cancer patients, 90
emotional aspects of illness
group therapy, 150
support, need for, 147, 149
Spiritual growth, 218–219
"Spirituality and Healing in Medicine"
(continuing education course),
121
Spontaneity, loss of, 136
Spouses and significant others, effect of
chronic illness on relationship,
164–176
body image and, 170
caregivers, need for support, 172–173
change, acknowledgment of, 174–175
communications between, 173–174
dating, 171–172
dreams, lost, 169
financial impact of illness, 167–169
frustration, dealing with, 167
fun, importance of, 175–176, 181
losses, grieving, 173
professional help, seeking, 175
relationship contract, renegotiating,
164–165
role reversals, 165–166
sexual relations, 169, 170
SSA: *see* Social Security Administration
(SSA)
SSDI: *see* Social Security Disability Insurance (SSDI)
SSI: *see* Supplemental Security Income
(SSI)
SSRIs: *see* Selective serotonin reuptake inhibitors (SSRIs)
Stanford University, 119
School of Medicine, 147
Psychosocial Treatment Laboratory,
90
Stereotypes, created by media, 143–144

Steroids, 79–80
Stress and chronic disease
biochemical changes, stress and, 44–
45
biological programming, stress and,
46
cause of illness, 29
definition of stress, 43–44, 253
emotional stressors, 40–41
fight-or-flight response, 43, 250, 253
general adaptation syndrome, 44
immune system stressors, 42–43
physical stress and, 41–42
postexertional malaise, 45
The Stress of Life (Selye), 43–45
Substance P, 253
Sulfa, 81
Superintendent of Documents
address, 262
Supplemental Security Income (SSI), 211
Supplements: *see* Herbs and supplements
Support and support groups, 147–156
caregivers, need for support, 172–173
cyberspace
caregivers, for, 172
evaluation of information, 154
flaming, 153, 250
interstitial cystitis, 23, 255
isolation, decreasing, 152–153
Lyme disease, 258
mailing lists, 151–152
newsgroups, 151–152, 252
spamming, 153–154, 253
Web sites, 151–152, 254
face-to-face support, 147–149
finding support group, 149–150
physician, ongoing support by, 61–62
psychotherapy, 150–151
twelve-step programs, 121, 145, 150
wellness groups, 150–151
Surgery
postponing, 67
unnecessary, 7
Swank, Roy L., 114
Swedo, Susan, 35
Sympathetic nervous system, 253
Symptoms: *see* Diagnosis; *specific illness*
Syndrome, defined, 254
Systemic lupus erythematosus
defined, 12, 254
depression, co-occurrence of, 35